# Ecological Risk of Persistent Pollutants in Kerala Estuaries

**Shaik Mohammad Hussain**

# Copyright © [2023]

**Title:** Ecological Risk of Persistent Pollutants in Kerala Estuaries

**Author:** Shaik Mohammad Hussain

This book was printed and published by [Publisher's Shaik Mohammad Hussain] in [2023]

ISBN:

For permission to reproduce any of the material in this book.

**CHAPTER - V**          **64**

## List of Tables

## List of Figures

# ABSTRACT

The present work is emphasized to demarcate the ecological risk status and delineate the environmental pollution factors from the surface sediments of the selected estuaries (Kadinamkulam, Anchuthengu, Kappil – Hariharapuram and Kayamkulam) along the south west coast of Kerala, India. Totally hundred and eleven surface sediment samples (Kadinamkulam - 23 samples; Anchuthengu - 32 samples; Kappil and Hariharapuram - 27 samples; Kayamkulam - 29 samples) were collected using Van Veen grab sampler, adopting the grid sampling technique. Various persistent pollutants such as trace elements, microplastics (MPs) and Polycyclic Aromatic Hydrocarbons (PAHs) were subjected to determine the ecological risk status from the sediments in the selected estuaries in Kerala. Sedimentological parameters such as sand-silt-clay ratio, calcium carbonate and organic matter in the sediment samples were determined. Trace element geochemistry and environmental pollution indices calculations were carried out by adopting standard methodologies. Forty-four sediment samples were chosen for the microplastics study and twenty sediment samples were selected for PAHs analysis.

Silt, sandy-silt and sand were the main sediment substrate in the selected estuaries. Silt is the dominant sediment observed in the estuary. Silty sediments deposit under calm waters and where the currents are weaker. Slightly higher concentrations of organic matter observed in the surface samples may be due to the adsorption and incorporation of organic materials from the overlying water column. The sediment samples were subjected to acid digestion technique for analyzing the following trace elements: Zn, Cu, Pb, Ni, Co and Cr. The total concentrations of the elements were measured using Atomic Absorption Spectrometry (AAS). The impact of anthropogenic activity is dealt with various environmental pollution indices. The distribution of the Fe and Mn was lower than the upper continental crust average (UCC) and local background concentration. The other elements like Pb, Zn, Co, Ni, Cr, and Cu in the sediments were less than the upper continental crust average (UCC) values. Anthropogenic impacts chiefly control the levels of PLI of the sediments. The study based on the SPI shows that sediments in selected estuaries ranges from natural sediments to highly polluted sediments. The grades of ecological risk of the metals suggest that in the selected estuaries majority of the sediment fall under the low-risk category.

The occurrence of the microplastics in sediments was due to the proximity of urban regions, distance of the sampling point from the coast. The mean abundance of the microplastic distribution in the sediments of selected estuaries was 628 particles/kg. The overall microplastics were dominated by coloured plastic, the size and shape classification suggest that they are conquered by < 1000 μm and fibre shape microplastic, respectively. The FTIR studies revealed that polyethylene, polyester and polypropylene were the dominant polymers among different types of microplastics in estuarine surface sediments. The potential ecological risk index values of selected estuarine sediments of the present study show extreme ecological risk from combined MP polymers in sediments. The analytical results of PAHs concluded that the surface sediments of the selected estuarine system falling under the low contamination and low-risk category. In this study, the ratio of LMW/HMW PAHs indicating that pyrolytic fractions dominate in these estuaries.

Based on the results from these proxies the overall risk status for the ecology of the selected estuaries is falling in low-risk status. As a sequel, few mitigative measures have also been suggested in order to cope up with the ecological risk aspects of these selected estuaries of the Kerala coast.

## ஆய்வுச் சுருக்கம்

இந்த ஆய்வானது, இந்தியாவின் கேரளாவின் தென்மேற்கு கடற்கரையில் உள்ள தேர்ந்தெடுக்கப்பட்ட முகத்துவாரங்களின் (கடினம்குளம், அஞ்சுதெங்கு, காப்பில் - ஹரிஹரபுரம் மற்றும் காயம்குளம்) மேற்பரப்பு வண்டல்களில் இருந்து சுற்றுச்சூழல் அபாய நிலையை வரையறுக்கவும், சுற்றுச்சூழல் மாசு காரணிகளை வரையறுக்கவும் வலியுறுத்தப்பட்டுள்ளது. வேன்-வீன் பிடி மாதிரியைப் பயன்படுத்தி, கட்ட முறை மாதிரி எடுத்தல் நுட்பத்தைப் பயன்படுத்தி மொத்தமாக நூற்று பதினொரு மேற்பரப்பு வண்டல் மாதிரிகள் (கடினம்குளம் - 23 மாதிரிகள்; அஞ்சுதெங்கு - 32 மாதிரிகள்; காப்பில் மற்றும் ஹரிஹரபுரம் - 27 மாதிரிகள்; காயங்குளம் - 29 மாதிரிகள்) சேகரிக்கப்பட்டன. கேரளாவில் தேர்ந்தெடுக்கப்பட்ட கரையோரங்களில் உள்ள வண்டல்களில் இருந்து சுற்றுச்சூழல் அபாய நிலையைத் தீர்மானிக்க, சுவடு கூறுகள் (Trace elements), நுண்நெகிழி (Microplastics) மற்றும் பல வளைய நறுமணமுள்ள நீரகக்கரிமங்கள் (PAHs) போன்ற பல்வேறு தொடர்ச்சியான மாசுபடுத்திகள் உட்படுத்தப்பட்டன. வண்டல் மாதிரிகளில் உள்ள மணல்-வண்டல்-களிமண் விகிதம், கால்சியம் கார்பனேட் மற்றும் கரிமப் பொருட்கள் போன்ற வண்டல் அளவுருக்கள் தீர்மானிக்கப்பட்டன. சுவடு உறுப்பு புவி வேதியியல் மற்றும் சுற்றுச்சூழல் மாசு குறியீடுகள் நிலையான முறைகளைப் பின்பற்றுவதன் மூலம் கணக்கிடப்படுகிறது. நுண்நெகிழி ஆய்வுக்காக நாற்பத்தி நான்கு வண்டல் மாதிரிகள் தேர்ந்தெடுக்கப்பட்டன மற்றும் PAH களின் பகுப்பாய்விற்கு இருபது வண்டல் மாதிரிகள் தேர்ந்தெடுக்கப்பட்டன.

தேர்ந்தெடுக்கப்பட்ட கழிமுகங்களில் வண்டல், மணல்-வண்டல் மற்றும் மணல் ஆகியவை முக்கிய வண்டல் அடி மூலக்கூறு ஆகும்.

வண்டல் என்பது முகத்துவாரத்தில் காணப்படும் முக்கிய வண்டல் படிவு வகை ஆகும். வண்டல் படிவுகள் அமைதியான நீரின் கீழ் மற்றும் நீரோட்டங்கள் பலவீனமாக இருக்கும் இடங்களில் படிகின்றன. மேற்பரப்பு மாதிரிகளில் காணப்பட்ட கரிமப் பொருட்களின் சற்று அதிக செறிவுகள், மேலோட்டமான நீர் நிரலிலிருந்து கரிமப் பொருட்களின் உறிஞ்சுதல் மற்றும் ஒருங்கிணைப்பு காரணமாக இருக்கலாம். வண்டல் மாதிரிகள் பின்வரும் சுவடு கூறுகளை பகுப்பாய்வு செய்வதற்காக அமில செறிமான நுட்பத்திற்கு உட்படுத்தப்பட்டன: Zn, Cu, Pb, Ni, Co மற்றும் Cr. தனிமங்களின் மொத்த செறிவுகள் அணு உறிஞ்சும் நிறமாலை (AAS) ஐப் பயன்படுத்தி அளவிடப்பட்டன. மானுடவியல் செயல்பாட்டின் தாக்கம் பல்வேறு சுற்றுச்சூழல் மாசு குறியீடுகளுடன் கையாளப்படுகிறது. Fe மற்றும் Mn இன் விநியோகம் மேல் கண்ட மேலோடு சராசரி (UCC) மற்றும் உள்ளூர் பின்னணி செறிவை விட குறைவாக இருந்தது. வண்டல்களில் உள்ள Pb, Zn, Co, Ni, Cr மற்றும் Cu போன்ற பிற தனிமங்கள் மேல் கண்ட மேலோட்ட சராசரி (UCC) மதிப்புகளை விட குறைவாக இருந்தன. மானுடவியல் தாக்கங்கள் முக்கியமாக வண்டல்களின் மாசுச் சுமை குறியிடு (PLI) அளவைக் கட்டுப்படுத்துகின்றன. வண்டல் மாசுக் குறியிடு (SPI) அடிப்படையிலான ஆய்வு, தேர்ந்தெடுக்கப்பட்ட கழிமுகங்களில் உள்ள வண்டல் படிவு வகை இயற்கை வண்டல்களிலிருந்து அதிக மாசுபட்ட வண்டல் வரை இருக்கும் என்பதைக் காட்டுகிறது. உலோகங்களின் சுற்றுச்சூழல் அபாயத்தின் தரங்கள் (PERI) தேர்ந்தெடுக்கப்பட்ட கழிமுகங்களில் பெரும்பாலான வண்டல் குறைந்த ஆபத்து வகையின் கீழ் வரும் என்று தெரிவிக்கின்றன.

வண்டல்களில் நுண்நெகிழி ஏற்படுவதற்கு நகர்ப்புறங்களின் அருகாமை, கடற்கரையிலிருந்து எழுவாயின் தூரம் காரணமாக இருந்தது. தேர்ந்தெடுக்கப்பட்ட கழிமுகங்களின் வண்டல்களில் நுண் நெகிழி

விநியோகத்தின் சராசரி மிகுதியானது 628 துகள்கள்/கிலோ ஆகும். ஒட்டுமொத்த நுண்நெகிழி வண்ண நெகிழி ஆதிக்கம் செலுத்தியது, அளவு மற்றும் வடிவ வகைப்பாடு அவை முறையே <1000 μm மற்றும் ஃபைபர் வடிவ நுண்நெகிழி மூலம் கைப்பற்றப்பட்டதாகக் கூறுகின்றன. ஃபோரியர் உருமாற்ற அகச்சிவப்பு நிறமாலை (FTIR) ஆய்வுகள், பாலி எதிலீன், பாலியஸ்டர் மற்றும் பாலிப்ரோப்பிலீன் ஆகியவை கழிமுகங்களில் மேற்பரப்பு வண்டல்களில் உள்ள பல்வேறு வகையான நுண்நெகிழிகளில் ஆதிக்கம் செலுத்தும் பாலிமர்கள் என்பதை வெளிப்படுத்தியது. தற்போதைய ஆய்வின் தேர்ந்தெடுக்கப்பட்ட கழிமுக படிவுகளின் சாத்தியமான சுற்றுச்சூழல் இடர் குறியீட்டு மதிப்புகள், வண்டல்களில் உள்ள ஒருங்கிணைந்த நுண்நெகிழி பாலிமர்களின் தீவிர சூழலியல் அபாயத்தைக் காட்டுகின்றன. பல வளைய நறுமணமுள்ள நீரகக்கரிமங்களின் (PAH) பகுப்பாய்வு முடிவுகள், தேர்ந்தெடுக்கப்பட்ட கழிமுக அமைப்பின் மேற்பரப்பு வண்டல்கள் குறைந்த மாசுபாடு மற்றும் குறைந்த-ஆபத்து வகையின் கீழ் வரும் என்று முடிவு செய்தன. இந்த ஆய்வில், LMW/HMW PAHகளின் விகிதம், இந்த கழிமுகங்களில் பைரோலிடிக் பின்னங்கள் ஆதிக்கம் செலுத்துகின்றன என்பதைக் குறிக்கிறது.

இந்த பதிலாள்களின் முடிவுகளின் அடிப்படையில், தேர்ந்தெடுக்கப்பட்ட கழிமுகங்களின் சூழலியலுக்கான ஒட்டுமொத்த இடர் நிலை குறைந்த ஆபத்து நிலையில் வருகிறது.

# CHAPTER - I
# INTRODUCTION

Pollutant denotes any particle or material that pollutes the environment by its presence. The source of these pollutants could be natural or artificial, but the artificial source is more prevalent than the natural source. The general pollutants are Heavy metals, Microplastics (MPs), phthalates, Polycyclic Aromatic Hydrocarbons (PAHs), Per Fluoro-alkyl substances (PFASs), pesticides, medical waste, microbes, fluoride etc. Pollution differs from contamination; however, contaminants can be pollutants and have a harmful effect on the environment. From literature, pollution is defined as the introduction by man, directly or indirectly, of substances or energy into the environment resulting in such deleterious effects as harm to living resources, hazards to human health, hindrance to environmental activities and impairment of quality for use of the environment and reduction of amenities. Contamination on the other hand is the presence of elevated concentrations of substances in the environment above the natural background level for the area and the organism. Environmental pollution can refer to undesirable and unwanted changes in physical, chemical and biological characteristics of air, water and soil which is harmful to living organisms both animals and plants. Pollution can take the form of chemical substances or energy, such as noise, heat or light (Wong, 2013). Pollutants, the elements of pollution, can either be foreign substances/energies or naturally occurring contaminants.

Persistent pollutants are toxic chemicals that adversely affect human health and the environment around the world. They are of greater global concern due to their potential for long-range transport, persistence in the environment, ability to bio-magnify and bio-accumulate in ecosystems, as well as their significant negative effects on human health and the environment. They can be transported through the atmosphere and water, most persistent pollutants generated in one country can and do affect people and wildlife far from where they are used and released. They persist for long periods in the environment and can accumulate and pass from one species to the next through the food chain.

Department of Geology, UNOM

## 1.1 TYPES OF POLLUTANTS

Environmental pollutants being a world concern, stand as one of the great challenges faced by the global society. The pollutants which cause adverse changes in the environment in contact can be naturally occurring compounds or live foreign matter. There are different types of pollutants, namely inorganic, organic and biological pollutants. The impacts, these pollutants bring into the environment have attracted a significant amount of attention, irrespective of the type of category they fall under. Environmental pollution and the world population show inarguable directly proportional relationship. As a result of the recent significant population growth, it is necessary to keep a keen watch on the amount of potentially harmful compounds released into the environment.

### 1.1.1 Inorganic pollutants

Inorganic pollutants contribute to the cause of adverse effects in the environment. The wastes produced by industrial, agricultural, and domestic activities that harm human and animal health are the sources of the aforementioned pollutant. Inorganic pollutants are usually substances of mineral origin, with metals, salts and minerals being examples (Wong, 2013). The reports from the studies profess the inorganic pollutants to be materials found naturally, that subsequently get their numbers increased in the environment by alterations made in the process of human production. Inorganic substances enter the environment through different anthropogenic activities such as mine drainage, smelting, metallurgical and chemical processes, as well as natural processes. These pollutants are toxic as a result of their accumulation in food chains (Salomons *et al.*, 2012).

### 1.1.2 Organic pollutants

Organic pollutants are biodegradable contaminants in an environment whose pollution sources are naturally found and caused by the environment. However, anthropogenic activity has also contributed to their intensive production in order to meet human needs. Some of the common organic pollutants which have been noted to be of special concern are human waste, food waste, polychlorinated biphenyls (PCBs), polybrominated diphenyl ethers (PBDEs), polycyclic aromatic hydrocarbons (PAHs), pesticides, petroleum and organochlorine pesticides (OCPs) (El-Shahawi *et al.*, 2010).

As a major problem in the environment, Organic pollutants grab greater attention and the properties of organic pollutants, amongst others, such as high lipid solubility, stability, lipophilicity and hydrophobicity have recently made organic pollutants termed as persistent. Such properties in organic pollutants cause toxicological effects, having the ability to easily bioaccumulate in the different spheres of the environment (Lepp, 2012; Van Ael *et al.*, 2012).

### 1.1.3 Biological pollutants

The existence of biological pollutants can be related to the flow of society and its impact on the quality of aquatic and terrestrial environments. This type of pollutant includes bacteria, viruses, moulds, mildew, animal dander and cat saliva, house dust, mites, cockroaches and pollen. The reports from the studies show various sources of these pollutants, including plants that produce pollen; people and animals carry bacteria and transmit viruses; bacteria held up by soil and plant debris (Elliot, 2003).

### 1.2 PERSISTENT POLLUTANTS CHOSEN FOR THE STUDY

There are numerous persistent pollutants in the environment. In the present study only three of the persistent pollutants are selected namely Heavy metals, Microplastics (MPs) and Polycyclic Aromatic Hydrocarbons (PAHs).

### 1.2.1 Heavy metals

Heavy metal has no specific definition but the description of heavy metal can be found in the literature. Heavy metal is a naturally occurring element that has a high atomic weight which is five times greater than that of water (Banfalvi, 2011). The toxicity of heavy metals makes it widely known among all the pollutants, receiving paramount attention from environmental chemists. Trace amounts of heavy metals are usually found in natural waters, even at very low concentrations, many of them are toxic (Herawati *et al.*, 2000). Metals such as arsenic, lead, cadmium, nickel, mercury, chromium, cobalt, zinc and selenium are highly toxic even in minor quantities. Highly alarming situation has been rising with a large number of industries dumping their metal effluents into freshwater without any appropriate primary treatments. The routine negligence of such industries has increased the number of metals in our resources (Salomons *et al.,* 2012).

Heavy metals, through food, water, air or absorption through the skin may enter the human body in agriculture, manufacturing, pharmaceutical, industrial or residential settings, and these substances are extremely toxic unless they are metabolized by the body and accumulated in soft tissues. Industrial exposure accounts for a common route of exposure for adults. Ingestion is the most common route of exposure in children. Even the natural and human activities discharge more than what the environment can handle, which ends up contaminating the environment and its resources (Herawati *et al.,* 2000; He *et al.,* 2005).

Heavy metals pollute the environment and its compartments. As a consequence, they have shrunk the ability of the environment to foster life and render its inherent values. These naturally occurring compounds are introduced in different environmental compartments by anthropogenic activities. The decline in the environment's ability to foster life threatens the health of humans, animals and plants. This occurs due to bioaccumulation of the non-degradable state of heavy metals subsisting in the food chain. Remediation of heavy metals requires special attention to protect all spheres of the environment such as the quality of soil, air and water, human and animal health, etc. The developed physical and chemical heavy-metal remediation technologies are expensive. Moreover, these time-consuming technologies come with drawbacks, releasing additional waste to the environment. Trace metals are mostly carried by the Sediments, as the metals are partitioned with the surrounding waters which reflect the quality of an environment. Heavy metals are persistent pollutants accumulating in organisms and bottom sediments in the coastal, estuarine and riverine regions (Szefer *et al.,* 1995).

The entire chemical composition of surficial sediments assesses the pathways by which the bottom sediments consisting of metals have accumulated, and it is considered a poor means of evaluation. But the same is regarded as a valuable index of environmental contamination. The non-detrital (non-residual) fraction of the total element is integrated into the sediments from the solution, whereas the detrital (residual) component forms the matrix of particles. Therefore, the determination of the chemical availability of metals on sediments is a way to find out the sources and pathways of major and trace elements entered into the marine environment (Loring and Rantala, 1992).

Heavy metals, as dissolved species in water or associated with suspended sediments, enter the riverine environment through natural and anthropogenic induced processes. The sediment incorporated metals can limit their bio-availability, remobilization and resuspension of sediments may return contaminants to the water column even when the external sources are eliminated (Al-Rousan *et al.,* 2016), however, multiple studies have connected sediment metal contamination to negative ecosystem impacts (Esslemont, 1999; Magesh *et al.,* 2011; Krishnakumar *et al.,* 2015; Magesh *et al.,* 2017). In addition, similar work was administered on sediments and water by various workers in other parts of the planet (Esslemont, 1999; Esslemont, 2000; Jayaraju *et al.,* 2009; Al-Rousan *et al.,* 2016).

## 1.2.2 Microplastics

Marine anthropogenic litter is an emerging pollutant of global concern. Several studies of recent years and international organizations around the world have highlighted the impacts caused directly and indirectly by its ubiquitous distribution. Microplastics harm aquatic ecosystems, marine animals, and local economies. Plastic is the most abundant fraction reported in international surveys, despite being made up of a variety of materials, with percentages varying from region to region. Microplastics (herein referred to as MPs) are a major source of concern in the plastics industry. Microplastics are plastic particles smaller than 5.0 mm in size (Arthur *et al.,* 2009). The lower bound (size) of the microplastics is not defined; however, it is common practice to use the mesh size (333 μm or 0.33 mm) of the Neuston nets used to collect the samples (Arthur *et al.,* 2009). There are two main ways microplastics are formed and enter a body of water: primary and secondary microplastics (Arthur *et al.,* 2009). The manufactured raw plastic material, such as virgin plastic pellets, scrubbers, and micro beds are the Primary microplastics (Browne *et al.,* 2007; Arthur *et al.,* 2009) that runoff from land to enter the ocean.

(Andrady, 2011). Secondary microplastic introductions occur when larger plastic items (meso- and macro-plastics) enter a beach or ocean and undergo mechanical, photo (oxidative) and/ or biological degradation (Thompson *et al.,* 2004; Browne *et al.,* 2007; Cooper and Corcoran, 2010; Andrady, 2011). Progressively smaller plastic fragments are formed through degradation, which breaks the larger pieces, and such smaller fragments are undetectable to the naked eye.

The anthropogenic contaminants present in almost all environments such as water, sediments, fishes and salt are microplastics. Scientifically it is a polymer made to fulfil our needs. They are natural sponges that absorb other contaminants around and also take a long time to degrade. This makes plastic wastes, highly hazardous contaminants. Plastic wastes demand huge environmental concern for they affect vast areas of land and aquatic environments due to their worldwide distribution. Recent researches have been giving more attention to plastics, which attributes to their longevity and long-distance distribution of plastics from their sources and accumulation in the global waters, including polar oceans (Thompson *et al.*, 2004; Cole *et al.*, 2011). Few recent studies have added information on MPs contamination in estuaries: Naidoo *et al.* (2015) reported the existence of MPs in five estuaries in South Africa while Zhao *et al.* (2015) studied MPs in three urban estuaries in China. Fok and Cheung (2015) have reported Pearl River as a potential source of MPs contaminating the estuary in Hong Kong to which the river joins. The occurrence and distribution of MPs in the surface water of the Three Gorges reservoir in China have been reported by Zhang *et al.* (2015). In the hydrological cycle, sediments are important carriers of trace metals. They are indicators of the quality of an aquatic system because metals are partitioned with the surrounding waters. The important sinks of these persistent pollutants are the coastal, estuarine and riverine regions.

### 1.2.3 Polycyclic aromatic hydrocarbons (PAH)

Polycyclic aromatic hydrocarbons (PAHs) are ubiquitous environmental pollutants. They are generated predominantly during incomplete organic material combustion. The organic materials include coal, oil, petrol and wood. Anthropogenic activities emit a major amount of PAH, but it cannot be ruled out that it could also be emanated from some natural sources such as open burning, natural losses or seepage of petroleum or coal deposits, and volcanic activities.

Major anthropogenic sources of PAHs include residential heating, coal gasification and liquefying plants, carbon black, coal-tar pitch and asphalt production, coke and aluminium production, catalytic cracking towers and related activities in petroleum refineries as well as and motor vehicle exhaust. PAHs are found in the ambient air in the gas phase and as a sorbet to aerosols. The fate of PAHs is influenced, from their transport in the environment to the way they enter a human body by atmospheric partitioning of PAH compounds between the particulate and the gaseous phases. The gas/particle partitioning strongly influences the removal of PAHs from the atmosphere using dry and wet deposition processes. Atmospheric deposition is a major source of PAHs in soil. Many PAHs have toxic, mutagenic and/or carcinogenic properties.

Polycyclic aromatic hydrocarbons are found in coal and tar deposits as uncharged, nonpolar molecules. Carbon and hydrogen, containing multiple aromatic rings, are the only contents of PAH. PAH possesses very characteristic UV absorbance spectra. Each isomer has a different UV absorbance spectrum, because of the unique UV spectrum of each ring structure. This makes it simpler to identify the PAH. They emit the characteristic wave lengths of light when they are excited and PAHs are mostly fluorescent in colour. PAHs are broadly pyrogenic or petrogenic in origin. The incomplete combustion of organic matter, for example, grass, wood, coal, petroleum and natural gas produce the pyrogenic PAHs (Lima *et al.,* 2003; Zhang *et al.,* 2015), while petrogenic PAHs are derived from crude oil and derivatives such as gasoline, diesel, lubricating oil, asphalt etc. (Ravindra *et al.,* 2008; Keshavarzifard *et al.,* 2014). PAHs associate so naturally with Aeolian/suspended particles that, they can easily transport through the atmosphere/water. This phenomenon is due to the hydrophobicity, low volatility and high persistence of PAHs (Ohkouchi *et al.,* 1999). PAHs transport to the estuarine and coastal systems majorly through direct input, river/urban runoff and atmospheric fall out including wet/dry deposition. (Parinos and Gogou, 2016). In the aquatic system, these compounds are attached to particulate matter and get deposited onto the sediment (Guzzella and De Paolis, 1994; Hu *et al.,* 2014) which may cause hydrocarbon contamination in the sediment; and, the consequent exposure to benthic biota might lead to acute/chronic toxicity (Weinstein *et al.,* 2010; Zeng *et al.,* 2013). Elaborate studies on the sources and the dynamics of PAHs were warranted as a result of rigorous assessment of potential hazards to the bio-resources.

The major PAH sources to the environment could be categorised into three types. They are: pathogenic, petrogenic, and biological. Whenever organic substances are exposed to high temperatures under low oxygen or no oxygen conditions, in the pyrolysis process, Pyrogenic PAHs are formed. The pyrolytic process can be conducted deliberately in the destructive distillation of coal into coke and coal tar, or the thermal cracking of petroleum residuals into lighter hydrocarbons. Meanwhile, other unintentional processes occur during the incomplete combustion of motor fuels in cars and trucks, the incomplete combustion of wood in forest fires and fire places, and the incomplete combustion of fuel oils in heating systems. The pyrogenic processes occur at temperatures ranging from about 350°C to more than 1200° C. The highest concentrations of pyrogenic PAHs are found in urban areas and areas close to major sources of PAHs. In addition, PAHs can also be formed at lower temperatures. It is worth mentioning that crude oils contain PAHs that formed over millions of years at temperatures as low as (100 – 150°C).

Crude oil maturation and similar processes are the means to form PAHs that are known as petrogenic. The widespread transportation, storage, and use of crude oil and crude oil products have made pathogenic PAHs very common. The oceanic and freshwater Oil spills, underground and above ground storage tank leaks and the accumulation of vast numbers of small releases of gasoline, motor oil, and related substances associated with transportation are recognized as the major sources of pathogenic PAHs. It is well-known that PAHs can be formed during the incomplete combustion of organic substances. PAHs are also found in petroleum products. On the other hand, it is not well-known that PAHs can be produced biologically. For example, certain plants and bacteria or degradation of vegetative matter can help to synthesize PAHs. The mode of PAHs formation can be either natural or anthropogenic.

## 1.3 STUDY AREA

Numerous estuaries and backwaters are connected with evenly urbanized inhabitants of Kerala along the west coast of the state. Geologically the Tertiary sediments cover Archean basement in the southern part of Kerala. Kallada, Karamaniyar, Vamanapuram, Ayiroor and Karipuzha are some major rivers that drain in these estuarine systems. Estuaries are highly polluted in areas where they occur. The direct discharge of fishing activities, industrial wastes, and sewage grains into estuaries has a greater impact on the quality of the water and contaminates the sediments in that area. Kerala is home to a vast body of brackish water known as backwaters, lakes, lagoons, and estuaries, as well as mangrove swamplands. The network of canals that facilitate the transport of men and material interconnect this chain of backwaters on the coastal plain. These backwaters have played a momentous role in the cultural and socio-economic history of Kerala. Mangroves are one of the most productive zones in the development of brackish water fisheries. Mangrove dependent or associated capture and captive fisheries and aquaculture is a notable feature of man-mangrove interaction, both biologically and economically. The detritus food web that provides rich food for several species of edible fin fish and shell fish is expanded throughout the mangrove ecosystem.

The four estuarine systems the selected for the present study in the southwest cost of Kerala are Kadinamkulam, Anchuthengu, Kappil- Hariharapuram and Kayamkulam (Fig. 1.1). The estuaries were selected based on the connectivity to the sea and the gap from the literature collected. In the present study, Kadinamkulam estuary located at southern sector when we move north, we have Anchuthengu, Kappil- Hariharapuram estuaries followed by Paravur estuary and Ashtamudi Kayal. Still further north locates Kayamkulam estuary. The accessibility to collect the samples from the Paravur estuary was associated with several issues and in the Ashtamudi Kayal there were number of researches carried already, so in the present study we choose the above-mentioned estuaries from south to north for better understanding of the persistent pollutants and its risk status.

**Kadinamkulam Kayal** (Lat 8° 35' to 8° 45' N and Lon. 76° 45' to 76° 56' E) in the Thiruvananthapuram district, one of the major retting zones dotting the coastal belt of Kerala, India was selected for this study. The Parvathyputhanar canal connects the Kayal to the Veli Kayal on the Southern part and the Anchuthengu Kayal on the northern part through the Vamanapuram River's lower reaches This is a temporary estuary and it has no direct connection with the Lakshadweep Sea, but we can witness seasonally through the opening of the sand bar at Perumathura, the connection of the two. During the present survey, the sand bar was closed.

Department of Geology, UNOM

**Anchuthengu Kayal** estuary near Chirayinkil in Thiruvananthapuram district. The Anchuthengu estuary meets with the sea through an inlet at Muthalapozhi and is almost parallel to the adjoining Lakshadweep Sea. There is a permanent opening to the sea for the estuary as a result of the construction of breakwaters. The Arabian Sea is seasonally connected to this estuary via the opening of the sandy bar. A temporary spit forms at the mouth for the rest of the year, rendering the estuary "blind." Natural conditions have changed as a result of the development of breakwaters and dredging works, allowing for continual mixing of fresh and sea water. The Vamanapuram River is the estuary's only source of freshwater.

**Kappil – Hariharapuram backwater** is a shallow brackish water system, which lies between 8°77'75.90" to 8°78'88.13"N latitudes and 76°67'58.48" to 76°67'68.83"E longitudes. Ayiroor Puzha is a small river that remains as the main freshwater inflow of this backwater system. The seventeen kilometres The Ayiroor Puzha begins in Navayikulam, Kerala's Midland region, and runs into the Edava Nadayara Kayal. The Ithikkara River, which begins in the Western Ghats and flows down to the Parvur Kayal, is another influence in the ecosystem of the Kappil backwaters. The lake's shores are shared between the districts of Kollam and Thiruvananthapuram. The Maniyamkulam canal connects it to Paravur Kayal. Here you can observe a natural Pozhi (bar mouth). The Kappil backwaters are connected to the Arabian sea by this natural Pozhi but a sand bar in the summer months splits the lake and the sea into two separate bodies. To promote tourism, the district tourism promotion councils of Kollam and Thiruvananthapuram manage two boat clubs, which provide tourists with boating amenities, generating revenue for the tourism industry. This backwater is frequently utilised for fishing, retting, relaxation, and aquaculture, among other activities. Some part of this backwaters where it is used for husk retting is contaminated and they secrete foul smell.

**Kayamkulam lake** is a narrow stretch of brackish water lying between 9°2'and 9°12'N latitude and 76°26' and 76°32'E longitude on the southwest coast of India. It offers great scope for aquaculture operations and is one of the best developed and little-explored estuarine habitats found in Kerala. During flood season freshwater canals empty water from the Pampa and Achankoil rivers into the lake. The tidal movements of the Arabian Sea influence the Lake through the Kayamkulam bar mouth which echoes in almost all parts of the lake. Ayirumthengu mangrove area is situated in the low-lying region on the southern portion of Kayamkulam Lake.

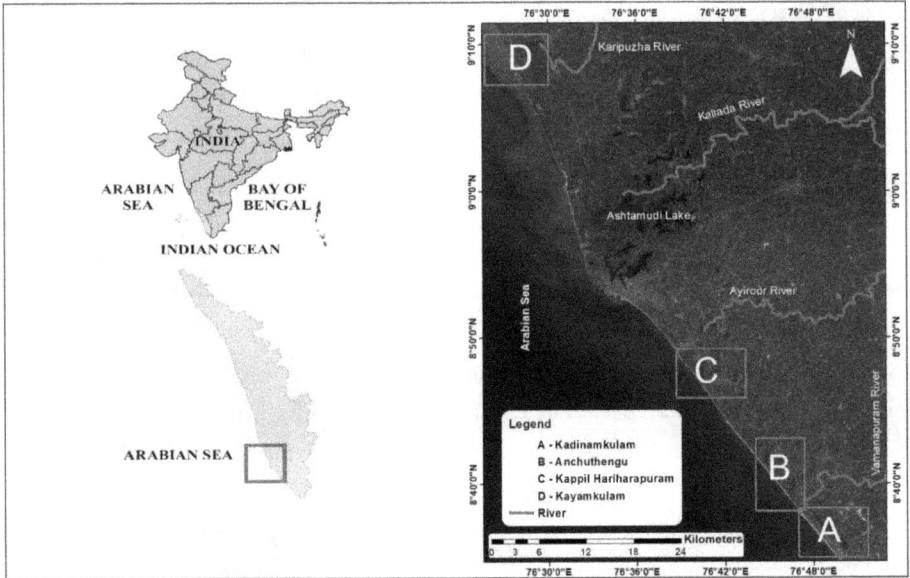

**Fig. 1.1** The study area map representing the selected estuaries in South west coast of Kerala, India

### 1.3.1 Climate

The Kayal area has seasonal heavy rain that influences the area to have a wet and maritime tropical climate. The annual mean temperature of this place ranges from a minimum of 25 °C (77 °F) to a maximum of 30 °C (86 °F). Humidity is higher in the mornings than in afternoons. A dry summer (pre-monsoon season) lasts from February to May, followed by the southwest monsoon season (June to September) with substantial rain and then the post-monsoon season (October to December) with low rainfall and few thunderstorms.

### 1.3.2 Temperature

Mean maximum temperatures are between 30° and 32°C in the coastal belts but go up to 38° C in the interior part of the watershed areas of the estuary. The seasonal and daily temperature changes are not consistent. The stations near the coasts are affected by land and sea winds, and their seasonal and diurnal temperature changes are nearly identical.

### 1.3.3 Rain Fall

Kerala does not experience continuous rains; instead, a few hours of rain are followed by sunny interludes that allow for the completion of all daily activities. Occasionally the rains might stretch on for a few days but sunshine is never far away. These golden interludes provide equilibrium to life's natural flow. Kerala has mainly two rainy seasons. The Southwest Monsoon that arrives in June is called Edavappathy. Mid-October witnesses the arrival of the Northeast Monsoon. The rain clouds gather from the Bay of Bengal and hurry to Kerala through the Palakkad Gap in the Western Ghats.

### 1.3.4 Hydrography

The chosen estuaries are shallow marginal lagoons with depths ranging from 0.4 to 3.4 metres. The estuary's salinity ranges from 25 to 31 PSU, and its temperature ranges from 31 to 34°C.

### 1.3.5 Geology

Kerala is one of the smallest states in India, located in the southwestern part of the Indian sub-continent bounded by northern latitudes 8°18' and 12°48' and eastern longitudes 74°52' and 77°22'. It is wedged in the east by the Western Ghats range and in the west by the Lakshadweep Sea, and covers an area of 38,863sq.km which forms 1.18% of the area of the Indian Union. Geologically, Pre-Cambrian crystalline rocks occupy the major part of Kerala. Sedimentary formations belonging to the Tertiary and Quaternary periods are fringed on the west of these crystalline rocks. The associations of various rock types, their stratigraphy along their mineralogy is briefly discussed.

The area surrounding the selected estuaries forms a major geological segment of the southern Indian peninsular shield. The area is covered by three major rock formations viz., the Archaean crystalline basement, the Tertiary and the Quaternary sedimentary sequences. In the eastern and southeastern regions of the river basins near the estuaries, the Archaean crystalline foundation is dominated by garnet–biotite gneisses, charnockites, and khondalites. The Quilon and Warkalli Formations are Tertiary deposits from the Lower Miocene period. Around the Sasthamkotta and Chelupola Lakes, the Warkalli Formation is exposed on laterite hillocks made of sandstones and clays. Fossiliferous limestones and sandy carbonaceous clays make up the Quilon Formation, which lies beneath the Warkalli Formation. The Archaean crystalline basement and the Tertiary sedimentary sequences are covered with the laterites. The Quaternary formations are epitomized by alluvial and sandy clays with peat. The main rocks are granite biotite gneiss with migmatite, Hornblende-gneiss Qz-felspatic-gneisses, charnockite, coastal sand, khondalite, laterite, quartzite, and sandstone.

## 1.4 OBJECTIVES OF THE PRESENT STUDY

The present research study from the estuaries of Kerala is undertaken with the following objectives.

➢ To discuss the textural characteristics and their depositional features.

➢ To estimate the estuarine system's possible ecological risk status based on heavy metals.

➢ To determine the risk status based on distribution and characterization of microplastics in the sediment substrate of estuarine sediments.

➢ To find out the carcinogenic potency, source and contamination of Polycyclic Aromatic Hydrocarbons (PAH) in the estuarine sediments.

# CHAPTER - II
# LITERATURE REVIEW

## 2.1 INTRODUCTION

Persistent pollutants are toxic chemicals that adversely affect human health and the environment around the world. They are of greater global concern due to their potential for long-range transport, persistence in the environment, ability to bio-magnify and bio-accumulate in ecosystems, as well as their significant negative effects on human health and the environment. They persist for long periods in the environment and can accumulate and pass from one species to the next through the food chain. Environmental pollutants being a world concern, stand as one of the great challenges faced by the global society. The pollutants which cause adverse changes in the environment in contact can be naturally occurring compounds or live foreign matter. There are different types of pollutants, namely inorganic, organic and biological pollutants. The impacts, these pollutants bring into the environment have attracted a significant amount of attention, irrespective of the type of category they fall under. As a result of the recent significant population growth, it is necessary to keep a keen watch on the amount of potentially harmful compounds released into the environment.

## 2.2 ENVIRONMENTAL PARAMETERS

Salinity induced gravitational circulation was the main reason causing the sedimentation in the estuary (Srinivas *et al.*, 2010). Distribution of sediment nature and rate of input are the major factors influencing the accumulation of sediments in estuary, shelf or coastal environment. Granulometric analysis have been commonly used in characterizing the sediment substrate in the shelf environment (Nittrouer *et al.*, 1983), transportation process and distribution of sediments in any area certainly affecting the bottom topography of recent environment (McCave, 1972). Being sensitive to environment, textural parameters analyses act as an indicator of the environmental condition (Koldijk, 1968). Numerous varieties of contaminants deposited and concentrated in the sediments of estuaries and the shelf floor due to rapidly increasing industrialization. Loring and Nota (1973) stated that calcium carbonate indicates the source of provenance and terrigenous materials dispersal pattern. Primary plankton, pollen, leaves and sewage residues possessing living organisms remains are the major sources of organic matter. Loring and Rantala (1992) stated that concentration of trace metals increases with reduction in grain size of the sediments, thus grain size parameters play an important role in geochemical studies. Organic matter has the ability to bind the trace metals and also carry those metals into diagenetic processes (Hunter and Liss, 1979; Balistrieri *et al.,* 1981). From the water column, the organic pollutants were removed by the sedimentation of the organic matter especially in association with the removal of the several trace metals (Mackereth, 1965; Pita and Hyne, 1975).

Muthusamy *et al.* (2021) estimated that majority of the sediments are silty sand and coarser in general in the Manakudy estuary. The center part of the estuary has silty sand indicating the influence of both marine and riverine characters. The mangroves growth in the center part of the estuary induces the microbial processes in OM decomposition leading to increase in finer sediment grains. Trend of $CaCO_3$ % in the estuary is low in the middle part and increasing towards the riverine and marine realms, shows positive correlation with sand percentage.

Hussain *et al.* (2020) reported the dominance of clayey substrate in the Ashtamudi estuary followed by sandy clay and clayey sand. Higher concentration of the organic matter (OM) was noted at the palm shaped arms of the lake as a result of high terrigenous input. Lower percentage of the OM was noticed at the middle part of the lake due to the constant seawater flushing through tidal cycles and by the confluence of Kallada river. The $CaCO_3$ is inversely proportional to organic matter. The higher percentage of the $CaCO_3$ is due to the presence of the shelled microfossils.

Saravanan *et al.* (2018) documented the sediment parameters in the Pulicat lagoon. Sandy and slity sand substrate are the dominant sediment substrate in the lagoon. Due to the confluence of the Kosasthalayar and Arani river southeastern part of the lagoon has predominance of the sandy substrate. Whereas the northwestern region of the lagoon has sandy silt and silt substrate due to the calm environment induced by the lack of freshwater influx by the ephemeral rivers. Due to high algal occurrence and shallow depth at the northwestern sector of the lagoon, higher percentage of organic matter was seen. Higher percentage of $CaCO_3$ was noted in the northwestern part of the lagoon due to the availability of shelled macro and micro-organisms.

Kalpana *et al.* (2016) studied the sediment parameters in the Uppanar estuary. The samples near to the estuarine mouth were sandy in nature with silt dominance in the upstream direction. The variation in sediment nature from location to location indicating the fluctuating discharge of river and estuarine influx. The area is dominated by sandy silt substrate. The higher value of organic matter was observed in the middle part of the estuary and in the mangrove regions. The lower content of $CaCO_3$ noted in middle part of the estuary and northern part due to gravity flow of sand as emplacement.

Jayaprakash *et al.* (2014) reported majority of the sediment substrate were clayey in nature at Ennore creek. Dominance of mud lead to the higher percentage of organic matter in the matrix. These results are due to the prevalence of weak flushing and calmer environment. The presence of carbonate content is inferred to be the product of underlying Tertiary limestones.

Hussain *et al.* (2013) documented the sediment parameters of the Ernakulam backwaters. Sandy and silty sand substrate in the backwaters of Ernakulam results in lower percentages of organic matter. Sand, sandy silt and silt are the dominant sediment substrate indicating relatively high energy environment.

Muraleedharan and Ramachandran (2002) studied the trace metal and textural aspects in Beypore estuary, Kerala. Upstream side has dominance of the sand whereas the sediment substrate show variation in the estuarine mouth with predominance of silt and clay. The major reason for fine grained sediments carried from the sea is flood tides.

## 2.3 TRACE ELEMENT GEOCHEMISTRY

Sediments have the ability to carry the elements and could behave as a sink for various contaminants in aquatic environments, particularly in marginal marine environment (Liu *et al.*, 2019; Herbert *et al.*, 2020). The estuarine and marine biota have a negative impact from the toxic elements existing in the aquatic environment (Nagarajan *et al.*, 2014; Islam *et al.*, 2017).

Physical, chemical and biological processes control the elemental concentration distribution in sediments (Ramanathan *et al.*, 1999; Selvam *et al.*, 2012). Even lower levels of toxic elements available to biological cycle are very harmful. There is a great need to understand the behavior of the trace elements distribution to encounter the problems in organisms by pollution. Heavy metals pollute natural environment becomes a global problem due to its persistence and their toxicity towards living organisms if they exceed their limit (Chakraborty *et al.*, 2009). Due to its abundance, persistence and environmental toxicity, trace element contamination in the estuaries attain global attention (Pekey, 2006; Ali *et al.*, 2016; Hwang *et al.*, 2016).

Cearreta *et al.* (2000) stated that the major source of pollutants along the marginal marine and marine environment was anthropogenic factors followed by natural weathering. The anthropogenic impact is felt strongly by coastal and estuarine environments lying adjacent to urban regions (Nouri *et al.*, 2008). Estuarine sediments were recognized to be the main entry point for pollutants into the ocean. Riverine metals generated from geogenic and anthropogenic sources are filtered by estuaries (Larrose *et al.*, 2010). In order to study the problem of metal contamination in coastal and estuarine environments rigorous investigations have been carried out to address its effects on biota and sediment profiles (Liu *et al.*, 2016; Jonathan *et al.*, 2016; Baran *et al.*, 2019). Effluent discharges from the urban areas and large industrial sites lead to the heavy metal accumulation in the estuaries and coastal environments (Ridgway and Shimmield, 2002). At the end of nineteenth century industrial revolution in Indian subcontinent markup the beginning of enrichment of trace metals in sediment profiles. In the aquatic environments, trace metals ultimately sink in the sediments. Hence, the history of the weathering pattern and metal accumulation of the sediments from nearby regions was reflected by the solid phase distribution in the sediments (Forstner and Salomons 1980; Nesbitt *et al.*, 1996).

Salam *et al.* (2021) studied threat to marine organisms and its effect to human health through degradation in the estuarine environment. The distribution of five trace metals (Cd, Pb, Cu, Fe and Zn) in the ten different estuaries at Kelantan, Malaysia was used to study the source, pollution level and potential risk status. Based on the inferences the dominant metal in the estuaries is Fe followed by Zn, Pb, Cu and Cu. The cluster analysis shows all the estuaries are almost polluted least by human influences. The estuarine surface sediments of Kelantan

Coastline based on the calculation of Geo-accumulation index (Igeo) exhibits polluted moderately by Fe and polluted strongly by Cd. Whereas the enrichment factor (EF) and ecological risk indices (RI) also exhibiting the similar results.

Liu *et al.* (2021) documented spatial distribution and characteristics of the heavy metal pollution in the surficial sediments of Haizhou Bay in China. Applying the Geo-accumulation index (Igeo) and the Hakonson pollution index were used to study the potential ecological risks based on seven trace metals. Trace element concentration was lower in the northern part whereas higher in the southern part of the Bay. Ranking of the heavy metals in the descending order of potential ecological risk index are Hg > Cd > As > Pb > Cu > Cr > Zn. Assessment of environmental quality show Hg is major heavy metal pollutant in the Bay. Various statistical factors were determined to correlate the trace metals and environmental elements, it shows consistent relation between the Igeo and the PERI.

Hussain *et al.* (2020) reported the environmental pollution status based on the heavy metal distribution of the Ashtamudi lagoon, Kerala. Eight heavy metals were employed to understand the heavy metal distribution and the potential ecological risk status. The north eastern part of the estuary shows low to moderate level of sediment pollution. The correlation analysis exhibits key role of fluvial input and natural weathering in the distribution of heavy metals in the estuarine surface sediments. Fe and Mn enrichment is controlled chiefly by fluvial process and enrichment of other studied elements are resulting from the anthropogenic influences. Accumulation of the trace elements mostly associated with finer fractions in the sediment substrate.

Saravanan *et al.* (2018) investigated the potential ecological risk index and sediment pollution index on the basis of trace element concentration from the 83 surface sediments of Pulicat lagoon, SE coast of India. Confluence of river and marine sources controls the textural characteristics, iron and manganese concentration in the estuarine surface sediments. Surface sediments are falling under less polluted based on sediment pollution index (SPI) and low potential ecological risk index category.

Magesh *et al.* (2017) have recognized the heavy metal pollution in the sediments at the nearshore province of the Tamiraparani estuary, Tamil Nadu. The sediments of the zone show high enrichment by Pb, significantly enriched by Ni and Co; moderately enriched by Cr. The Geo-accumulation index (Igeo) shows that the sediments are heavily polluted with Pb, moderately polluted with Co and Ni, and unpolluted with the remaining elements. Detrital components and heavy metals assigned to the finer portion of the sediment substrate are the sources of Fe and Mn in the sediment. In the southern part of the estuary concentration of the Ni is higher indicating the anthropogenic contamination by river discharge. Similarly in the northern part of the estuary higher concentration of the Pb noted as a result of industrial effluences from thermal power plant and also by port activities.

Salas *et al.* (2017) studied the pollution level status of the surficial sediments of Cochin estuary in Kerala using nine heavy metals (Fe, Mn, Zn, Cr, Pb, Ni, Co, Cu and Cd) as proxies. Based on various pollution indices studied, the northern arm of the estuary is severely enriched with trace element concentration. Correlation matrix show relation between metals, finer substrate and organic matter, since the finer substrate and organic matter were key carriers for the trace elements. Multivariate analyses imply Ni and Cu are derived from natural weathering process and enrichment of Cr, Cd, Pb and Zn were chiefly attributed to various anthropogenic activities.

Kalpana *et al.* (2016) reported the pollution status based on the heavy metal concentration and anthropogenic influences in the surface sediments at Uppanar estuary, Cuddalore, Tamil Nadu. NI, Cr and Cu show concentrations above the continental crust value indicating effluence from metal industries and surface runoff from the agricultural lands having higher fertilizer remain. Heavy metals show attribution of Fe and Mn through the adsorption on Fe-Mn oxyhydroxides. The area is polluted moderately by anthropogenic influences. Correlation factor shows positive relation between the trace elements and the organic matter. The Geo-accumulation index (Igeo) exhibits the sediments are unpolluted to moderately polluted concerning Fe and Cu, whereas with Pb and Co sediments falling under moderate to considerably polluted category. The study reveals anthropogenic activities are major sources of heavy metal contamination.

Department of Geology, UNOM

Muralidharan and Ramasamy (2014) investigated the distribution of trace element in the sediment core of Punnakayal estuary, Tamil Nadu. Most of the samples are dominated clayey silt substrate. Calcium carbonate and organic matter were increasing down the core. The heavy metal concentration is in decreasing order of the following metals Fe, Mn, Cr, Pb, Ni, Zn and Cd. Higher concentration of the heavy metals is resulting due to the anthropogenic effluences from nearby places industries.

Magesh *et al.* (2013) studied the trace elements based pollution status from the sediments in three estuaries (Kallar, Korampallam creek and Punnakayal) of Tuticorin coast, Tamil Nadu. In these estuarine sediments the enrichment factor and geo-accumulation index results show predominant pollution by As, Cd, Hg. As and Pb. The component factor investigation reveals the source of the heavy metal accumulation in the sediments. Fe and Mn are derived from the river sources and Hg and As derived from the untreated industrial sewages. Korampallam creek among other selected area show high contamination by trace elements as a result of discharge effluents from Tuticorin alkali chemicals, thermal power plant, copper smelting, shipping activities and Petrochemical industries.

Heavy metals, through food, water, air or absorption through the skin may enter the human body from agriculture, manufacturing, pharmaceutical, industrial or residential settings, and these substances are extremely toxic unless they are metabolized by the body and accumulated in soft tissues. Industrial exposure accounts for a common route of exposure for adults. Ingestion is the most common route of exposure in children. Even the natural and human activities discharge more than what the environment can handle, which ends up contaminating the environment and its resources (Herawati *et al.*, 2000; He *et al.*, 2005).

The entire chemical composition of surficial sediments assesses the pathways by which the bottom sediments consisting of metals have accumulated, and it is considered a poor means of evaluation. But the same is regarded as a valuable index of environmental contamination. The non-detrital (non-residual) fraction of the total element is integrated into the sediments from the solution, whereas the detrital (residual) component forms the matrix of particles. Therefore, the determination of the chemical availability of metals on sediments is a way to find out the sources and pathways of major and trace elements entered into the marine environment (Loring and Rantala, 1992).

Heavy metals, as dissolved species in water or associated with suspended sediments, enter the riverine environment through natural and anthropogenic induced processes. The sediment incorporated metals can limit their bio-availability, remobilization and resuspension of sediments may return contaminants to the water column even when the external sources are eliminated (Al-Rousan *et al.,* 2016), but several studies have linked sediment metal contamination to detrimental effects on ecosystems (Esslemont, 1999; Jayaraju *et al.,* 2009; Magesh *et al.,* 2011; Krishnakumar *et al.,* 2015; Al-Rousan *et al.,* 2016; Gopal *et al.,* 2017).

## 2.4 MICROPLASTICS

Marine anthropogenic litter is an emerging pollutant of global concern. Several studies of recent years and international organizations around the world have highlighted the impacts caused directly and indirectly by its ubiquitous distribution. Microplastics harm aquatic ecosystems, marine animals, and local economies. Plastic is the most abundant fraction reported in international surveys, despite being made up of a variety of materials, with percentages varying from region to region. Microplastics are plastic particles smaller than 5.0 mm in size (Arthur *et al.,* 2009). There are two main ways of microplastics are formed and enter a body of water: primary and secondary microplastics (Arthur *et al.,* 2009). The manufactured raw plastic material, such as virgin plastic pellets, scrubbers, and micro beds are the Primary microplastics (Browne *et al.,* 2007; Arthur *et al.,* 2009) that runoff from land to enter the ocean. (Andrady, 2011). Secondary microplastic introductions occur when larger plastic items (meso-and macro-plastics) enter a beach or ocean and undergo mechanical, photo (oxidative) and/ or biological degradation (Thompson *et al.,* 2004; Browne *et al.,* 2007; Cooper and Corcoran 2010; Andrady, 2011). Microplastics (herein MPs) are a major source of concern among polymeric products because of their ability to adsorb persistent, bio-accumulative, and toxic chemicals (PBTCs) and trace elements under weathering conditions (e.g. solar radiation, water temperature, and abrasion processes) (Frias *et al.,* 2018).

Ranjani *et al.* (2021) reported an early review on the ecological risk status of various environments in India based on the microplastics. Researchers are interested in the abundance, chemical characteristics, and ecological risk of microplastics (MPs) in terrestrial and aquatic ecosystems. This is the first approach to know the ecological danger of MPs in sediments throughout the Indian coast using meta-data. Sediment quality was assessed using the polymer hazard index (PHI), pollution load index (PLI), and potential ecological risk index (PERI). Places with high PHI values (>1000) have high hazard scores owing to the influence of polymers with high hazard scores, such as polyamide (PA) and polystyrene (PS). MPs are moderately contaminated in sediments along India's west coast (WCI) (PLI: 3.03 to 15.5), while sediments on India's east coast (ECI) are far less contaminated (PLI: 1 to 6.14). The PERI values of sediments throughout the Indian coast revealed that metropolitan towns, river mouths, and strong hydropower plants, potential fishing zones, and remote islands were at higher ecological risk.

Xu *et al.* (2020) documented he microplastics in sediment samples collected from Liaohe estuary and its two main inflowing rivers were analyzed. FT-IR was used to identify and confirm the presence of 19 different types of polymers in sediment samples, including the three most common polymers (polyethylene, polyethylene terephthalate). These microplastics occur in four different shapes, with percentages ranging from high to low: film, fragment, fibre, and pellet. Microplastics were found in lower abundance in river sediments from the Shuangtaizi River, with an average of 170±96 particles/kg d.w., compared to the Daliao River, which had an average of 237±129 particles/kg d.w., but it was higher than in the Liaohe Estuary, which had an average of 120± 46 particles/kg d.w. Furthermore, the highest concentrations of microplastics were discovered near river mouths, indicating a high accumulation where freshwater and saltwater meet.

Patterson *et al.* (2020) focussed on the presence and characteristics of microplastics (MPs), as well as the spatial distribution and pollution status of heavy metals in the water and sediments of coral reef ecosystems associated with the Tuticorin and Vembar groups of islands in the Gulf of Mannar, southeast India. Mean abundance of MPs varies from 60±54 to 126.6±97 items/L in water and from 50±29 to 103.8± 87 items/kg in sediment. Water and sediment samples from the Tuticorin islands contain higher MP concentrations than the Vembar islands.

The mainland samples had the highest MP, while MP distributions in the shoreward direction, i.e., towards the islands, closely mirrored those of the mainland (p0.05). Polyethylene is the most common polymer, with fibres (1-3 mm) being the most common form in water and fragments (3-5 mm) being the most common in sediment.

Veerasingam *et al.* (2020) reviewed the scientific literature on microplastic (MP) pollution in India's diverse environmental matrices and to identify research gaps for upcoming research objectives The origins, distribution, transport pathways, destiny, impacts, chemical hazards, and MP organisms relationships in India's fresh water and marine ecosystems were all assessed, as well as the current methodologies for sampling, extraction, identification, characterization, and quantification of MPs. Few research has been done on MPs' spatial and temporal transport pathways, especially in relation to stream flow, anthropogenic factors, beach morphology, bottom topography, biofouling, and hydraulics.

Alves and Figueiredo (2019) reported microplastics distribution in Gunbara Bay, Brazilian coast. Microplastics were separated and classified according to their type, colour, size, and polymer composition. Microplastic abundances (160 to 1000 items/kg or 4367 to 25,794 items m2) were high regardless of area or period, indicating that microplastics are abundant in Guanabara Bay. The translucent polyester microfiber with a diameter of 1mm was the most abundant microplastic in the sediment; this is a secondary microplastic that could have come from washing machine waste. When compared to the majority of studies conducted around the world, the extremely high availability of microplastics in Guanabara Bay suggests a high risk of contamination to benthic organisms and demersal fish, as they may be ingesting microplastics.

McEachern *et al.* (2019) studied to measure the abundance and distribution of microplastics in surface waters and sediments in Tampa Bay, Florida. The concentrations of microplastics in discrete water samples ranged from 0.25 to 7.0 particles/L, with an average of 0.94 (0.52) particles/L. 1.2–18.1 particles/m3 were found in samples taken with a 330 m plankton net, with an average of 4.5 (2.3) particles/m3. Discrete samples were 200 times more-higher than net samples, implying significant losses or under sampling with the net. There were no significant differences in concentrations between stations or regions for both discrete and plankton tow samples. Summer rainfall events were always preceded by samples with significantly higher counts. The majority of microplastics (more than 75%) were fibres. Tampa Bay contains 4 billion microplastic particles based on an average value of 1 particle/L. Surface sediments had an average particle density of 280 (290) particles/kg, with a range of 30 to 790 particles/kg. Microplastic concentrations were highest in sediments near industrial sources; lowest values in Middle and Lower Tampa Bay are consistent with shorter residence times.

Mukhanov *et al.* (2019) reported the microplastics occurrence and distribution in Sevatopol Bay, Black Sea. The traditional NOAA protocol for MP extraction from seawater was combined with a simple and inexpensive method for analyzing the shape and size spectrum of all MP particles in the sample in this pilot study. For image acquisition, a standard flatbed scanner with a slide adapter was used, and MP dispersive properties (particle abundance, shape, and size spectrum) were quantified using Image software. For the particle analysis, Feret's diameter and circularity (or roundness) appeared to be the most efficient shape descriptors. In terms of abundance and mass, the first reliable estimates of MP concentrations in Black Sea coastal waters (Sevastopol Bay) accounted for 0.6 to 7 items m-3 and 6 to 750 g m-3, respectively. There are no steady-state gradients in MP distribution along the transect from the bay's mouth to its corner. MP inflow to bay waters and transport along the bay appeared to be controlled by a complex combination of factors including rainfall, wind regimes, currents, and Black River discharge.

Gray *et al.* (2018) investigated microplastic distribution in the intertidal sediments of Charleston Harbor and Winyah Bay, both in South Carolina, the average particle concentration was 413.8 76.7 and 221.0 25.6 particles/m2, respectively. The average particle concentration/L in the sea surface microlayers of Charleston Harbor and Winyah Bay was 6.6 1.3 and 30.8 12.1, respectively. The concentration of microplastics in the two estuaries' intertidal sediments was not significantly different (p=0.58), but Winyah Bay contained significantly more microplastics in the sea surface microlayer (p=0.02). While, microplastic concentration in these estuaries was comparable to that reported for other estuaries worldwide, Charleston Harbor contained a high abundance of black microplastic fragments believed to be tire wear particles.

Lithner *et al.* (2011) provided an elaborate methodology to assess the microplastic based risk status of on environment. Plastics are a large material group, with global annual production more than doubling in the last 15 years (245 million tonnes in 2008). Plastics are ubiquitous in society and the environment, particularly in the marine environment, where massive amounts of plastic waste accumulate. Human and environmental hazards and risks from chemicals associated with a wide range of plastic products are poorly understood. The majority of chemicals used in the production of plastic polymers are derived from nonrenewable crude oil, and several of them are hazardous. These may be emitted during the manufacturing, use, and disposal of the plastic product. The environmental and health risks of chemicals used in 55 thermoplastic and thermosetting polymers were identified and compiled in this study. For the hazard classes and categories in the EU classification and labelling (CLP) regulation, which is based on the UN Globally Harmful Substances List, a hazard ranking model was developed. Initial assessments were made after ranking the polymers based on monomer hazard classifications. The polymers ranked as the most dangerous are composed of mutagenic and/or carcinogenic monomers (category 1A or 1B). Polyurethanes, polyacrylonitriles, polyvinyl chloride, epoxy resins, and styrenic copolymers are examples of polymer families. Each has a sizable global annual production (1–37 million tonnes). A significant number of polymers (31 out of 55) are composed of monomers from the two lowest of the ranking model's five hazard levels, namely levels IV–V. Phenol formaldehyde resins, unsaturated polyesters, polycarbonate, polymethyl methacrylate, and urea-formaldehyde resins are polymers made of level IV monomers with a large global annual production (1–5 million tonnes). This study identified hazardous substances used in polymer production whose risks should be assessed before deciding whether risk reduction measures, substitution, or even phase out are required.

Microplastics (MPs) are widely acknowledged as a global emerging threat to aquatic ecosystems and biodiversity. Despite the fact that the number of publications and interest in MP research has increased rapidly, it is still difficult to compare the obtained data due to the use of different methodologies in MP assay. As a result, there is an urgent need for a standardized approach to MP quantification procedures in order to produce comparative assessments.

## 2.5 POLYCYCLIC AROMATIC HYDROCARBONS (PAHs)

PAHs (polycyclic aromatic hydrocarbons) are common contaminants in the environment. They are generated predominantly during incomplete organic material combustion. The organic materials include coal, oil, petrol and wood. Anthropogenic activities emit a major amount of PAH, but it cannot be ruled out that it could also be emanated from some natural sources such as open burning, natural losses or seepage of petroleum or coal deposits, and volcanic activities. Major anthropogenic sources of PAHs include residential heating, coal gasification and liquefying plants, carbon black, coal-tar pitch and asphalt production, coke and aluminium production, catalytic cracking towers and related activities in petroleum refineries as well as and motor vehicle exhaust. PAHs are found in the ambient air in the gas phase and as a sorbet to aerosols. The fate of PAHs is influenced, from their transport in the environment to the way they enter a human body by atmospheric partitioning of PAH compounds between the particulate and the gaseous phases. The gas/particle partitioning strongly influences the removal of PAHs from the atmosphere using dry and wet deposition processes. Atmospheric deposition is a major source of PAHs in soil. Many PAHs have toxic, mutagenic and/or carcinogenic properties.

The major PAH sources to the environment could be categorized into three types. They are: pathogenic, petrogenic, and biological. Whenever organic substances are exposed to high temperatures under low oxygen or no oxygen conditions, in the pyrolysis process, Pyrogenic PAHs are formed. The pyrolytic process can be conducted deliberately in the destructive distillation of coal into coke and coal tar, or the thermal cracking of petroleum residuals into lighter hydrocarbons. Meanwhile, other unintentional processes occur during the incomplete combustion of motor fuels in cars and trucks, the incomplete combustion of wood in forest fires and fire places, and the incomplete combustion of fuel oils in heating systems. The pyrogenic processes occur at temperatures ranging from about 350°C to more than 1200° C. The highest concentrations of pyrogenic PAHs are found in urban areas and areas close to major sources of PAHs. In addition, PAHs can also be formed at lower temperatures. It is worth mentioning that crude oils contain PAHs that formed over millions of years at temperatures as low as (100 – 150°C).

Polycyclic aromatic hydrocarbons are found in coal and tar deposits as uncharged, nonpolar molecules. PAHs are broadly pyrogenic or petrogenic in origin. The incomplete combustion of organic matter, for example, grass, wood, coal, petroleum and natural gas produce the pyrogenic PAHs (Lima *et al.,* 2003; Zhang *et al.,* 2015), while petrogenic PAHs are derived from crude oil and derivatives such as gasoline, diesel, lubricating oil, asphalt etc. (Ravindra *et al.,* 2008; Keshavarzifard *et al.,* 2014). PAHs associate so naturally with Aeolian/suspended particles that, they can easily transport through the atmosphere/water. This phenomenon is due to the hydrophobicity, low volatility and high persistence of PAHs (Ohkouchi *et al.,* 1999). PAHs transport to the estuarine and coastal systems majorly through direct input, river/urban runoff and atmospheric fall out including wet/dry deposition. (Parinos and Gogou, 2016).

Li *et al.* (2021) studied distribution and pollution of PAHs from the sediments in ten estuaries of China. Anthropogenic influences attribute complex sources of PAHs and its increasing distribution in estuarine environment. Economic size and human population were used to illustrate the anthropogenic impacts on PAHs contamination in estuaries. The total PAHs concentration ranging from 60.9 – 330.7 ng/g in wet season and from 103.9 – 620.6 ng/g in dry season across the estuaries. The concentration of the total PAHs at the continental scale reveals higher proportion at dry season than wet season. There is a significant correlation between total PAHs concentration and per capita GDP across the estuaries. The chief source of PAHs were biomass combustion and coal-processing as indicated by the $\delta 13C$. The results reveal increasing anthropogenic activities intensified thus increases the total PAHs pollution in the estuarine sediments.

Rajan *et al.* (2019) investigated occurrences and sources for the major 16 PAHs in the sediments of two urban rivers Adayar and Cooum in Chennai city. The results of the study reveals that the low molecular weight (LMW) PAHs are lesser than the high molecular weight (HMW) PAHs. The HMW PAHs prevalence indicates the incomplete combustion. The emission source for the PAHs were pyrogenic and some significant part from petrogenic sources revealed from the principal component analysis. The informal recycling of e-wastes and industrial effluences were the possible sources for the presence of high molecular weight PAHs. The effect estimation by ecological risk assessment suggesting the PAHs cause slight adverse effect to no effect in both the rivers except few locations that are affected by e-waste sites and residential sites having moderate to heavy ecological impact.

Rajpara *et al.* (2017) assessed the PAH exposure, toxicological indices and its effect in the Gulf of Kutch region, Gujarat. Total concentration of PAHs ranges from 118280 – 1099410 ng/g dw with abundance of low molecular ring PAHs comparing to high molecular ring PAHs. The concentration level of carcinogenic and mutagenic PAHs was ranging from 8120 – 160000 ng/g dw, it is higher than acceptable limit. The toxicological profile of this study has significance since it has a lot of information regarding the pollutants like PAHs and the methods to manage with higher concentrations in least explored marine environments.

Ramzi *et al.* (2017) reported the distribution and occurrence of PAHs in the Cochin estuary, Kerala, SW coast of India. PAHs in the estuarine sediments reveal seasonal dynamics. The concentration level of PAHs ranging from 304 to 14149 ng/g. The estuary sediments were substantially contaminated by LMW PAHs, which increased at a quicker rate during the monsoon, suggesting river/land runoff as a major transportation mechanism. The predominance of the LMW PAHs reveals the combustion at lower temperature and petrogenetic sources and low levels of the HMW PAHs indicating the lesser contribution from the pyrolytic sources. The values of carcinogenic toxicity equivalents (TEQ) calculated show it ranges from 1 – 971 ng/g in the surficial sediments.

Masood *et al.* (2016) applied PAHs as anthropogenic markers for the organo-chemical pollution in the estuarine sediments of the Selangor River, Malaysia. The total PAHs concentration ranging from 203 – 964 ng/g dw. The level of PAHs is higher in the wet season comparing to the dry season indicating the domestic sewage discharge and higher urban runoff taking the pollutants from nearby areas. The Sediment Quality Guidelines (SQGs) applied to measure the toxic contaminants concentration, and the results reveals that the PAHs levels were under the SQGs. Thus, it would not affect the biota adversely.

Sanil Kumar *et al.* (2016) studied seasonal and spatial distribution of the PAHs in the sediments of the Chitrapuzha River, Kerala, India. During the season of pre-monsoon higher level of PAHs exists due to some point sources of PAHs situated in the industrial zones along the river course. Based on the n-Alkaline indices and the diagnostic PAHs ratio show the petroleum contamination in the surface sediments. The detected concentration of the PAHs in the sediments reveals the capability of the contaminants to cause negative impact on biota.

Pérez-Fernández *et al.* (2015) documented homologues of PAHs in the marine sediments along the Galician ria, Ría de Arousa, Spain. Pressurized Liquid Extraction (PLE) method and gas chromatography coupled to mass spectrometry (GC–MS) was adapted to extract and quantify the PAHs. The concentration of the total PAHs ranges from 44.8 – 7901 ng/g dw. The sediments retrieved near the harbour show highest concentration of PAHs and at the outer region of ria were noted as cleanest positions from PAHs.

Jaward *et al.* (2012) reported distribution and occurrence of PAHs in water, sediment and some biota of Estero de Urias estuary in Mexico. The most dominant PAHs in the studied sediment samples was Phenanthrene followed by pyrene and naphthalene. The concentration of the total PAHs ranges from 27 – 418 ng/g. The contamination sources are mainly attributed by anthropogenic activities like industrial and domestic discharges, street runoff and vehicle emissions. The higher concentrations of the PAHs were noted in the rainy season. The results from the toxicity tests reveals that the PAH concentration could be dangerous to several aquatic organisms especially during their early growth stages.

Essien *et al.* (2011) studied the distribution of the PAHs in sediments from Iko River estuary, Nigeria. The PAHs ranges from 6.10 – 35.27 mg/kg dw. The benthic sediments have higher capacity to act as a sink for accumulating chemical pollutants. The results show the sources are from industrial sewages through runoff and biogenic origin. The origin of the PAHs is from pyrolytic sources with little impact of petrogenic sources.

Garcia *et al.* (2010) documented distribution of the PAHs in sediments from the Patos Lagoon estuary, Southern Brazil. Sediments lying near the City of Rio Grande noted to be contaminated by PAHs by urban discharge effluence. According to the sources the effluents were clustered into 4 groups namely industrial, sewage, runoff and mixed, representing various

Department of Geology, UNOM

contribution of PAHs. Among these runoff and mixed sources were predominant. The maritime navigation and related actions were second major PAHs source to sediments. The origin of the PAHs was identified as pyrolytic basically. Uncontrolled dumping and accidental discharge of PAH was noted at some locations lying nearer to the gas stations and automobile workshops.

Zhang *et al.* (2004) reported occurrence of PAHs and its persistence, toxic effects from various matrix including water, pore water, soil, sediment and vegetables from Minjiang River Estuary in China. The PAHs ranges from 112 – 877 ng/kg dw. The contamination was dominated by HMW PAH compounds indicating sources derived from combustion (high temperature pyrolysis). The selected PAHs ratios reveals the source for the PAHs were derived mainly from partial combustion of hydrocarbons/fossil fuels.

# CHAPTER - III

# MATERIALS AND METHODS

This chapter discusses the many techniques used in sample collecting, processing, and analysis (Flow chart. 3.1).

## 3.1 FIELDWORK

Grid sampling technique and Van Veen grab sampler were used to collect a total of 111 surface sediments (Fig. 3.2) from estuaries of southwest Kerala coast (Kadinamkulam - 23 samples (A); Anchuthengu - 32 samples (B); Kappil and Hariharapuram - 27 samples (C); Kayamkulam - 29 samples (D)) during April - 2019. For sediment characteristics and trace element geochemistry, Zip lock covers were used to preserve the samples and they were additionally secured with rubber bands to ensure no sample loss. The zip lock covers were properly labeled as each sample was placed in them. For microplastics study, the samples were transferred into the pre-cleaned glass bottles and for PAHs, using a pre-clean stainless-steel spatula, collected surface sediment was transferred to amber-colored glass jars and stored in the icebox. As soon as the fieldwork was over, the samples were immediately taken to the geochemical laboratory, University of Madras and carried out further studies.

## 3.2 SEDIMENT CHARACTERISTICS

Organic matter, calcium carbonate, Sediment texture, and trace metals analyses were carried upon the sun-dried surface samples. Exothermic heating and oxidation with potassium dichromate and concentrated $H_2SO_4$, followed by titration of excess dichromate with 0.5N ferrous ammonium sulphate solutions, were used to assess the organic content (Gaudette *et al.,* 1974). The procedure of (Piper, 1947) was used to determine and calculate the calcium carbonate ($CaCO_3$) content. Sand, Silt and Clay distributions (Krumbein and Pettijohn, 1938) were determined for the textural studies of the sediments.

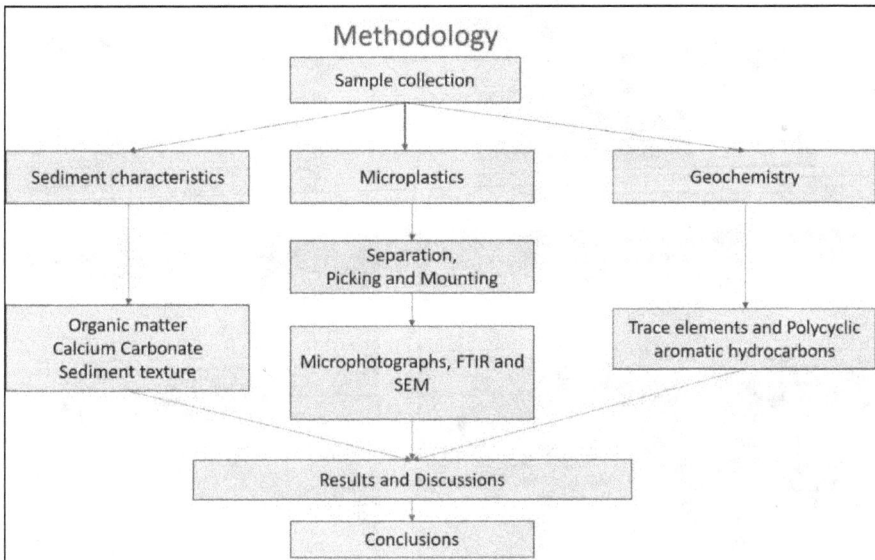

**Fig. 3.1** Flowchart representing the methodology for various analyses adapted in the present study

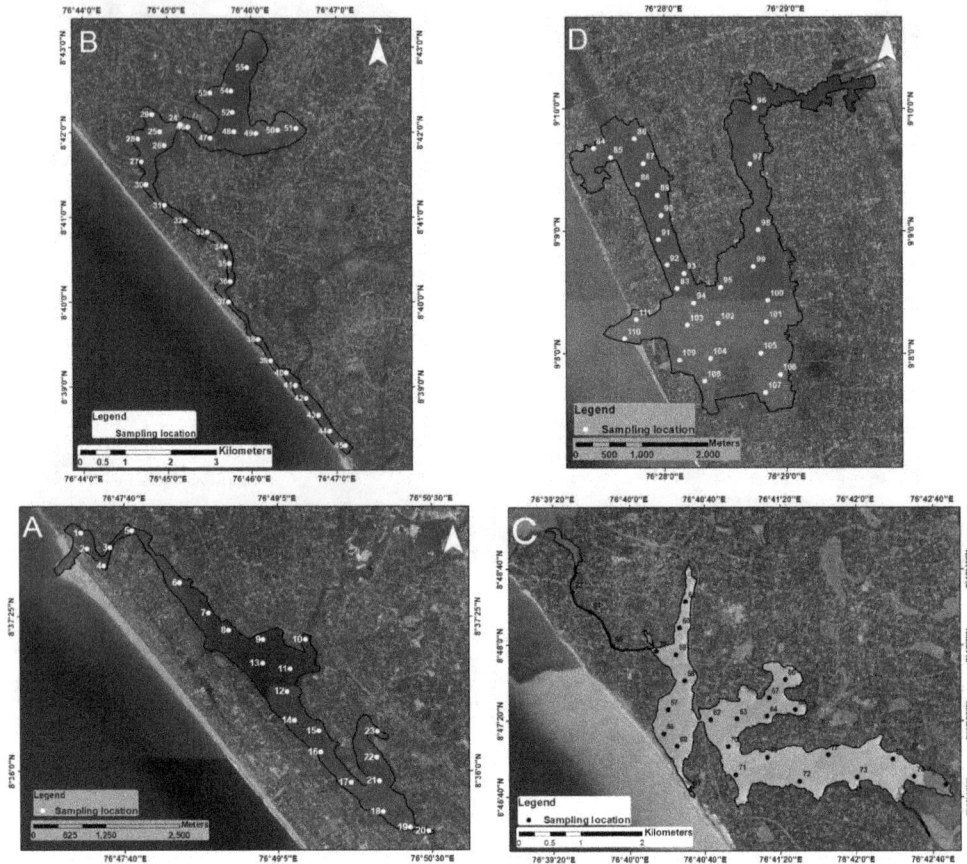

**Fig. 3.2** Map representing the sampling locations from the selected estuaries,

southwest coast of Kerala, India

## 3.2.1 Determination of Calcium Carbonate

Carbonate is generally a crucial component of marine sediments. It is considered to be a vital indicator of the source area and dissemination of the continental terrestrial materials in the Gulf of St. Lawrence (Loring and Nota, 1973). In the current study, the rapid titration method (Piper, 1947) was used to determine the calcium carbonate content. Since the values of carbonates other than calcium carbonate are insignificant, for practical purposes the total carbonate is referred to as calcium carbonate in the present analysis.

### Procedure

The following procedure was followed for the determination of the calcium carbonate content in the surface sediments: 150 ml beaker is taken and 5.0 g of the sediment is weighted and shifted into the beaker. A pipette with an enlarged jet is used to measure and pour 100 ml of 1N hydrochloric acid into the beaker. A watch glass is placed on the beakers to cover its mouth and aggressively stirred multiple times for one hour. When the solution is settled, with the help of a pipette 20 ml of supernatant liquid is pipetted out into a small Erlenmeyer flask. 6-8 drops of bromothymol blue indicator are added to the pipetted liquid and titrated against sodium hydroxide solution. For certain samples, the indicator colour might vanish indicating the endpoint and blue colour is observed. When this happens, more indicator is added and the titration is completed. To determine the titre value of hydrochloric acid, a blank titration is performed. The below equation can be used to calculate the calcium carbonate percentage.

*Percentage of calcium carbonate = (Blank titration - Actual titration) x 5*

### 3.2.2 Determination of readily oxidisable Organic Matter

To identify the part played by the organic component of the sediments in transport & deposition, organic matter is determined. The Walkey-Black method, as outlined by Jackson (1958) is used to identify the easily oxidizable organic carbon content. This process is used to separate the humus matter from extraneous sources or organic carbon such as graphite or coal. This procedure is considered in the present study because Gaudette *et al.* (1974) identified that this technique provided exceptional accordance with the LECO combustion method of organic carbon analysis. The Walkey-Black method makes use of oxidation and exothermic heating with concentrated sulphuric acid and potassium dichromate of the samples, followed by the titration of excess dichromate with 0.5 N ferrous ammonium sulfate solution to a precise, one drop end point. Silver sulfate can be used in the digestion mixture to prevent the oxidation of chloride in the digestion mixture.

## Procedure

The dried sediment sample is sieved using a 230 microns sieve; 500 ml Erlenmeyer flask is taken and 0.5g of the sieved sample is put in the flask. Burette is used to measure out precisely 10 ml of 1 N potassium dichromate solution and 20 ml of concentrated sulphuric acid with silver sulfate which are added to the flask and are mixed by slowly rotating the flask for a minute. The mixing of the contents with the sample is done with utmost care to ensure that there is no sediment on the sides of the flask out of reach from the reagents. After allowing the mix to rest for 30 minutes, add 10 mL of 85 percent orthophosphoric acid and 0.2 g sodium fluoride. Later 15 drops (0.5 ml) of the diphenylamine indicator are added to the sample flask. The final solution is titrated against 0.5 N ferrous ammonium sulfate solution. The titration is conducted to a precise one-drop brilliant green endpoint. As the titration continues, the colour of the mixture advances from an opaque greenish-brown to green upon the addition of around 10 ml of the ferrous solution. The colour continues to change with titration to a bluish-black grey. Now, the introduction of 10-20 drops of the ferrous solution changes the colour to a brilliant green giving one drop endpoint. With each new batch of sediment samples, a standardization blank without sediment is run and recorded.

## Calculation of results

$$\text{\% Organic Matter (readily oxidisable)} = 10 \ (1 - T/S) \times F$$

Where,

   S = standardisation blank titration, ml of ferrous solution

   T = sample titration, ml of ferrous solution

   F = factor derived as follows:

   $F = (1.0 \ N) \times 12/4000 \times 1.72 \times 100/\text{sample weight}$

    (1.03, when sample weight is exactly 0.5 g)

Where,

   12/4000 = meq wt. carbon and

   1.72 = factor for organic matter from carbon.

Department of Geology, UNOM

### 3.2.3 Determination of Sand, Silt and Clay ratio

Shallow water sediments are generally composite types comprising of particles within the size range from sand to clay with their dissimilar combinations.

### Procedure

To remove the moisture content, all base sediment samples are entirely dried in a hot air oven. The disaggregated sample is washed through a 230 ASTM sieve (mesh opening = 0.063 mm) until spotless water passes through, keeping in mind that the washings do not exceed 1,000 ml. The sample preserved on the sieve is made to dry. It is then weighed to determine the sand fraction. With the help of the pipette method following the procedure adopted by Krumbein and Pettijohn (1938), the fine fraction (silt and clay) is examined. The suspension passing through the sieve is gathered in a 1 litre graduated measuring cylinder. If the suspension is less than 1,000 ml after thorough washing, the already prepared sodium hexametaphosphate solution is added to bring it up to 1,000 ml.

The suspension in the measuring cylinder is disturbed well using a stirrer to have same distribution of the particles in suspension. The time when the stirring was stopped is noted, and precisely after 2 hours and 3 minutes, a 20 ml pipette is slowly placed in to a depth of 10 cm in the solution and the sample is withdrawn with uniform suction to avoid any disturbance. The pipetted-out sample is transported to a 50 ml beaker which is pre-weighed. It is carefully dried in an oven, avoiding boiling and splashing. The weight of the clay particles is calculated from the weight of the beaker leftovers after all of the liquid and moisture content has dried. By subtracting the consolidated weight of the sand and clay fragments from the measured sample weight, the weight of the silt fragments is estimated. The sand, silt, and clay fragments' individual weights are converted to weight percentages and shown on a trilinear diagram. Trefethen's (1950) textural nomenclature is used to describe the sediments in the present study.

### 3.3 TRACE ELEMENT GEOCHEMISTRY

The bulk sediment was mixed and a homogenised mixture was made by means of the cone and quartering method to determine the trace element content. The sediment fractions were obtained by passing the homogenised mixture through the 230 ASTM mesh after it had been

Department of Geology, UNOM

ground with an agate mortar. The ground sediments were then sealed in airtight containers for further geochemical examination. A Teflon bomb with a closed stainless-steel jacket assembly was used to digest the silt. Below is a detailed technique for the entire digestion approach. The acid combination (HNO3: HClO4: HF - 4:3:2 ratio) was applied to 0.5 g of crushed fine-grained particles (<63 μm) in the Teflon beaker, then the digesting assembly was suitably locked and placed in the hot plate for two hours. The temperature of the hot plate was sustained at 120°C (Hussain *et al.,* 2020). The digestion assembly was allowed to cool after the digestion process, and the final solution was filtered and made up with 50 mL of deionized double distilled water. The made-up solution was kept in conventional plastic vessels for elemental analysis. The elemental analysis was accomplished with the help of a Graphite Furnace Atomic Absorption Spectrophotometer (Model no - Perkin Elmer-PinAAcle 900AA) at Department of Geology, University of Madras, Chennai. In the instrument configuration, double replication was maintained, and the mean value was used as the final output for further analysis.

### 3.3.1 Computation of Pollution Indices

Various methods to find out the heavy metal contamination and categorize by quantitative indexes were tried to deduce the anthropogenic input from the geo-genic input.

### 3.3.1.1 Enrichment Factor (EF)

EF was determined to discover if the metal levels in the sediments of selected estuarine sediments and its surrounding marine environment were of anthropogenic origin (e.g., contamination). Various authors have successfully utilized Fe to normalize heavy metals contaminants. In the present study also, Fe was adopted as a conservative tracer to distinguish natural from anthropogenic components. According to Ergin *et al.* (1991), the metal EF is defined as follows:

$$EF = \frac{(M/Fe)_{Sample}}{(M/Fe)_{Background}}$$

Where,

M – Metal concentration of the sediment

The classification of enrichment classes was:

> ➤ If, EF < 1 indicates no enrichment (natural enrichment),
>
> ➤ If, EF 1-3 for minor enrichment,
>
> ➤ If, EF 3-5 for moderate enrichment;
>
> ➤ If, EF 5-10 for moderately severe enrichment,
>
> ➤ If, EF 10-25 for severe enrichment,
>
> ➤ If, EF 25-50 for very severe enrichment, and
>
> ➤ If, EF >50 for extremely severe enrichment.

### 3.3.1.2 Geo-accumulation Index (Igeo)

The geo-accumulation index was originally defined by Muller (1969). Despite the fact that Igeo was designed to be used using worldwide regulatory shale data as background metal levels, Rubio et al. (2000) found that using regional background values produced more meaningful findings. Geo-accumulation index (Igeo) can evaluate the extent of the pollution process (Muller, 1979). Igeo calculation was accomplished only for the surface sediment in each core.

$$I_{geo} = \log_2 (C_n / 1.5 * B_n)$$

Where,

Cn is the heavy metal content in the sediment that has been measured.

$B_n$ is the geochemical background value in average shale (Turekian and Wedepohl, 1961) of element n

1.5 is the background matrix correction in factor due to litho-genic effects.

To evaluate the sediment quality, Muller specified the following ranges. $I_{geo}$ value and Sediment Quality ranges were as follows

> ➤ If $I_{geo}$ < 0, Unpolluted;
>
> ➤ If $I_{geo}$ 0-1, From unpolluted to moderately polluted;
>
> ➤ If $I_{geo}$ 1-2, Moderately polluted;
>
> ➤ If $I_{geo}$ 2-3, From moderately polluted to strongly polluted;
>
> ➤ If $I_{geo}$ 3-4, Strongly polluted;
>
> ➤ If $I_{geo}$ 4-5, From strongly to extremely polluted;
>
> ➤ If $I_{geo}$ >5, Extremely polluted.

Department of Geology, UNOM

### 3.3.1.3 Contamination Factor (CF)

Hakanson (1980) had suggested a contamination factor (CF) and the degree of contamination ($C_d$) to describe the contamination of toxic substance.

$$CF = C_{metal} / C_{background}$$

Where,

CF - contamination factor

$C_{metal}$ - concentration of pollutant in sediment

$C_{background}$ - background value for the metal

CF values indicate the enrichment of metals in the sediments.

 ➢ From $1 \leq CF$ low contamination factor

 ➢ If $1 \leq CF < 3$ moderate contamination factor

 ➢ If $3 \leq CF < 6$ considerable contamination factor

 ➢ If $\geq 6$ very high contamination factor

### 3.3.1.4 Pollution Load Index (PLI)

Tomlinson *et al.*, 1980 had followed a simple approach based on the Pollution Load Index (PLI) to estimate the degree of pollution by metals in estuarine sediments. Sediment PLI was calculated using the equation.

$$CF = C_{metal} / C_{background}$$

$$PLI = n (CF1 \times CF2 \times CF3 \times \text{........} \quad CFn)$$

**Where,**

CF - contamination factor

$C_{metal}$ - concentration of pollutant in sediment

$C_{background}$ - background value for the metal

n - number of metals

**PLI status:** PLI > 1 polluted; < 1 no pollution

### 3.3.1.5 Potential Ecological Risk Index (PERI)

Hakanson (1980) proposed a potential ecological risk index. PERI uses ecological analysis to assess the impact of heavy metals on the ecosystem (Guo et al., 2010; Saeedi et al., 2012). The following formulae can be used to compute the risk index (RI).

$$C_f^i = C_D^i / C_B^i$$

$$E_r^i = T_r^i \times C_f^i$$

$$RI = \sum_{i=1}^{m} E_r^i$$

Here, RI is the sum of individual heavy metal potential risks, $E_r^i$ is the individual heavy metal potential risk, $T_r^i$ is the toxic-response factor for a selected metal (Hakanson, 1980), Cf I is the contamination factor, $C_D^i$ is the current concentration of metals in sediments, and $C_B^i$ is the background concentration record of metal in crust (Taylor, 1964). Hakanson (1980) divided the ecological risk (Ei) grades into five categories and the potential ecological risk index (RI) into four categories.

Ecological risk grades are as follows

| *Ei* | - | *Ecological risk level* |
|------|---|-------------------------|
| < 40 | - | Low |
| 40 – 80 | - | Moderate |
| 80 – 160 | - | Considerable |
| 160 – 320 | - | High |
| $\geq$ 320 | - | Very high |

Potential ecological risk index (RI) grades are as follows

| *RI* | - | *Ecological risk level* |
|------|---|-------------------------|
| < 150 | - | Low |
| 150 – 300 | - | Moderate |
| 300 – 600 | - | Considerable |
| $\geq$ 600 | - | High |

### 3.3.1.6 Sediment Pollution Index (SPI)

Singh et al. (2002) suggested the sediment pollution index SPI as a way to assess sediment quality in terms of trace metal concentration and metal toxicity. The SPI can be denoted as:

Department of Geology, UNOM

$$SPI=\sum \frac{EFm \times Wm}{\sum Wm}$$

$$EF_m = \frac{Cn}{CR}$$

Here, Wm is the toxicity weight, and EFm is the ratio between the measured metal concentration (Cn) and the background metal concentration (CR). According to Hakanson (1980), Cr and Zn have a toxicity weight of 1, Cu and Ni have a toxicity weight of 2, Pb has a toxicity weight of 5, and Cd has a toxicity weight of 30. Based on this pollution classification, the SPI was classified as following:

➢ From 0 to 2 = natural sediment,

➢ From 2 to 5 = low polluted sediment,

➢ From 5 to 10 = moderately polluted sediment,

➢ From 10 to 20 = highly polluted sediment, and

➢ Greater than 20 = dangerous sediment.

## 3.4 MICROPLASTIC SEPARATION

The homogenized surface sediment samples were carefully placed in glass bottles with a metal lid to avoid contamination. The wet samples were sieved through a 5 mm mesh to preserve particles of <5 mm size and eliminate larger debris. The sediment was shifted to ceramic bowls and placed in the hot oven at 60°C. The oven-dried samples were homogenized and then passed through the 5 mm testing sieve to eliminate the coarse debris and organic plant remains (Sruthy and Ramasamy, 2017). National Oceanic and Atmospheric Administration (NOAA) protocol (Masura *et al.*, 2015) was taken into account for the extraction of MPs from sieved sediment samples. Therefore, 30g of dried sediment was treated with 30% Hydrogen peroxide ($H_2O_2$) solution followed by 2N HCl to remove the organic matter and calcareous phase from the surface sediments. Next, the density separation method was done as follows: The pre-treated estuarine sediments were completely mixed with 50 ml of pre-prepared zinc chloride solution (density: 1.58 g/cm3). The mixture was filtered using 0.45 μm Whatman® nitrocellulose membrane filter paper and vacuum pump assembly. Filtration was done three times for better extraction results. The filter paper was analyzed under an optical stereo zoom microscope for microplastic distribution. The shape of the retained particles above filter paper was classified (Free *et al.,* 2014) as a fibre (thin or fibrous, straight plastic particle), film (thin plane of flaky plastic particle), pellet/beads (hard, rounded plastic particle), and fragment (hard, jagged plastic particle).

The separated polymer compositions were identified using the Bruker Fourier-Transform Infrared Spectroscopy (FTIR) method in combination with the Attenuated Total Reflectance (ATR) diamond crystal attachment. The microplastic compositions frequency curve was identified using a readily available spectral library with instrument setup. The extracted microplastic was classified based on the colour, shape, and composition of the materials under the optical stereo zoom microscope in Polarizing mode with an online digital camera setup (Model – NIKON SMZ25). The microplastic distribution in terms of colour, shape, size, and composition were depicted in the pie chart. The graphical illustrations were prepared using the Microsoft Excel software package (Microsoft office, 2007).

### 3.4.1 Risk assessment of MPs in sediments

Microplastics along the additives used with them often known as cocktail of contaminants, persistent organic pollutants and heavy metals exist in the environment (Rochman, 2015). The mixture of microplastics with its additives can be bioavailable to numerous biota and humans through ingestion (Hartmann *et al.,* 2017). As a result, it's critical to analyse the ecotoxicological risk of MPs in order to have a clear picture of the potential harm when they're consumed by biota. Unreacted monomers and hazardous additives remain while synthesizing the MPs from a chain of monomers by polymerization process. MPs in the beach and sea surface emit toxic chemicals as a result of thermal breakdown and photo degradation. Plastics with chemical components more than 50% are classified as hazardous by the United Nations' Globally Harmonized System of categorization and labelling of chemicals (Lithner et al., 2011; Rochman et al., 2013). Results based on the ecological risk assessment of MPs in the sediments has not received much attention. Using Polymer Hazard Index (PHI) and Potential Ecological Risk Index (PERI) as the parameters the ecological risk assessment of MPs in estuarine, marine and terrestrial sediments is assessed.

### 3.4.2 Polymer Hazard Index (PHI)

To assess the possible dangers of MPs in surface sediments, we observed at both their concentration and chemical composition as stated by Xu *et al.,* 2018. Chemical toxicity of various polymer kinds of MPs is examined when assessing ecological impact (Lithner *et al.,* 2011). The following formula was used to calculate the polymer hazard assessment of MPs:

$$PHI = \Sigma Pn \times Sn$$

where 'PHI' stands for the computed polymer hazard index induced by MP, 'Pn' stands for the proportion of specific polymer types collected at each sampling location, and 'Sn' stands for the hazard scores of MP polymer types derived from Lithner *et al.,* 2011.

### 3.4.3 Potential Ecological Risk Index (PERI)

The Potential Ecological Risk Index (PERI) is used to determine the extent of MPs contamination in sediments (Peng et al., 2018). The equations used to calculate the PERI are as follows:

$$Cif = Ci/Cin$$

$$Ti\ r = \Sigma^n_{n=1}\ Pn\ /Ci \times Sn$$

$$Eir = Tir \times Cif$$

where, Ci is the concentration of pollutant 'i' (i.e., microplastic) and Cin is the concentration of unpolluted samples. Toxicity and biological sensitivity are represented by the toxicity coefficient (Tir). The toxicity coefficient is calculated by multiplying the percentage of particular polymers in the entire sample (Pn/Ci) by the plastic polymer hazard score (Sn) (Table. 3.1).

**Table. 3.1** Representing the various Hazard score based on MPs

| PHI | Hazard category | PERI | Risk category |
|---------|-----------------|----------|---------------|
| 0-1 | I | <150 | Minor |
| 1-10 | II | 150-300 | Medium |
| 10-100 | III | 300-600 | High |
| 100-1000 | IV | 600-1220 | Danger |
| >1000 | V | >1200 | Extreme |

## 3.5 POLYCYCLIC AROMATIC HYDROCARBONS

Using a pre-clean stainless-steel spatula, the surface sediment was transferred to amber-colored glass jars and stored in the ice box. The sediments were immediately transported to the laboratory and maintained in a deep freezer at -20°C until they were analysed. The samples were given to CVR Labs P. Ltd, Saidapet, Chennai, India for PAHs analysis.

During the extraction of the PAH fraction, the sonication/ultrasonic agitation method was applied to achieve greater extraction efficiencies (Sun *et al.,* 1998). As a result, the freeze-dried and homogenised sediment was utilised to extract the PAH using a dichloromethane – methanol (2:1) solvent mixture in a sonication/ultrasonic agitation bath for 48 hours, and the resulting extract was treated with activated granular copper to remove sulphur impurities. Finally, the extract was purified using the silica-alumina (2:1) column cleanup method after the extracted solution was evaporated using the rotary evaporation method. The aliphatic compounds were then removed from the column by eluting it with n-hexane. The column was then eluted with n-hexane to remove the aliphatic compounds, followed by a combination of n-hexane and dichloromethane to remove the PAH compounds (3:7 ratio). The near-dryness extract was prepared for PAH detection using 500 μl n-hexane after the final extract was evaporated by a moderate nitrogen stream. A flame ionisation detector on an Agilent 7890B Series Gas Chromatograph was used to evaluate sixteen PAHs listed by the USEPA. The temperature of the column for analyses was set to 60°C (starting time, 2 minutes) at a rate of 10°C per minute, then to 120–300°C at a rate of 3° C per minute, and finally to 310° C for 5 minutes. During both injection modes, the injector and detector were kept at 280° C and 325° C, respectively, and the injection volume was 2 L. On the basis of the recovery output of a known amount of PAH reference combination, the extraction efficiency was double-checked. PAH recovery rates ranged from 82 percent to 95 percent. All chemical analyses were performed in triplicate, and the output values were represented in dry weight.

### 3.5.1 The Toxic Equivalent (TEQ)

The total amount of potentially carcinogenic PAH congers in the sediment was used to determine its toxicity range (TCPAH - BaA, Chr, BbF, BkF, BaP, DbA, and InP fractions; Chen and Chen, 2011). The TCPAH levels in the estuarine surface sediments ranged from 16 to 44.21

ng/g. The TCPAH analytical result was lower than the ERL-ERM levels reported by SQGs (1373– 8410 ng/g; Long *et al.,* 1995). The toxic equivalent (TEQ) of each PAH was calculated using the equation below (Nasher *et al.,* 2013; Li *et al.,* 2015).

$$Total\ TEQ = \sum_i Ci \times TEFi$$

Toxicity factor (TEFi) of the individual fractions, and Ci is the concentration of an individual PAH fraction. BaA, Ch, BbF, BkF, BaP, IP, and DbA have TEFs of 0.1, 0.001, 0.1, 0.01, 1, 0.1, and 1 (Roesner and Traina, 1994).

### 3.5.2 Source of the PAHs

PAH sources can be identified using the ratio of low molecular weight to high molecular weight PAH components. The estimated ratio greater than 1 denotes a petrogenic source of PAH, whereas the ratio less than 1 denotes a pyrolytic source.

# CHAPTER - IV
# TEXTURAL CHARACTERISTICS AND DEPOSITIONAL ENVIRONMENTS

## 4.1 SEDIMENT TEXTURE

In order to understand the ecological conditions, environmental parameters have been analyzed from the collected sediment samples. Salinity induced gravitational circulation was the main reason causing the sedimentation in this estuary (Srinivas *et al.,* 2010). Distribution of sediment nature and rate of input are the major factor influencing the accumulation of sediments in estuary, shelf or coastal environment. Granulometric analysis have been commonly used in characterizing the sediment substrate in the shelf environment (Nittrouer *et al.,* 1983), transportation process and distribution of sediments in any area certainly affecting the bottom topography of recent environment (McCave, 1972). Being sensitive to environment, textural parameters analyses act as an indicator of the environmental condition (Koldijk, 1968). Numerous varieties of contaminants deposited and concentrated in the sediments of estuaries and the shelf floor due to rapidly increasing industrialization. The sediment texture has important role in controlling the concentration of the pollutants in the sediments, where the level of pollutant concentration increases with decreasing particle size. To determine and assessing the influence of the anthropogenic sources in the sediments it is necessary to know the effect of the grain size of the sediments or geochemistry (Zhang *et al.,* 2007).

### 4.1.1 Kadinamkulam

The Kadinamkulam estuary has no direct connection with the Arabian Sea, however it is connected with the Sea through an opening at Perumathura seasonally. During the sample collection, the sand bar was closed. The relative abundance of sand, silt and clay in the surface sediments of Kadinamkulam estuary has been estimated (Table 4.1). Sand content ranges from 0.6 percent to 89.4 percent with an average of 30.6 percent, silt content from 10.2 to 98.8% with an average of 69.0 percent, and clay content from 0 to 0.8 percent with an average of 0.4 percent in the studied region (Fig. 4.1). The maximum percentages of sand fraction have been found in northern part of the estuary especially the estuarine mouth and the southern part of the estuary connecting to the Veli kayal through Parvathy puthanar canal. From the observations the higher proportion of sand is a result of wave and tide-controlled sedimentation in the estuarine mouth and the fresh water influx in the southern part. Silt is the dominant sediment observed in the estuary. Whereas the presence of clay substrate even though least dominant substrate has enrichment at center of the estuary indicates the calm environment due to lack of freshwater influx and confluence of the transient streams into the estuary. Similar observation was found in Uppanar estuary, where sandy silt is dominant sediment substrate (Kalpana *et al.*, 2016).

### 4.1.2 Anchuthengu

The sand, silt and clay ratio in the surface sediments of Anchuthengu has been estimated (Table 4.2). In the study area, Sand content extends from 0% to 95.8%, with an average of 39.4 percent; silt content goes up to 99.6%, with an average of 60.1 percent; and clay content is from 0% to 5%, with an average of 0.5 percent. (Fig. 4.2). The inferences from the spatial distribution map, the proportion of sand is higher in the sediments along the connecting canal of the Anchuthengu estuary and the Kadinamkulam estuary having the confluence of the lower reaches of Vamanapuram River with these estuaries. Silt is the dominant sediment substrate in the estuary indicating the calm environment prevailing there. Along the direction of downstream, trend of decreasing in grain size is observed. This is resulting from the differential transportation mechanism of the river, which in turn controlled by velocity of water and seasonal variation (Yasin *et al.*, 2016).

### 4.1.3 Kappil and Hariharapuram

Kappil and Hariharapuram estuaries were connected to Paravur kayal by Maniyamkulam canal. In Kappil and Hariharapuram estuaries, the relative abundance of sand, silt and clay in the sediments of surface sample has been estimated (Table. 4.3). In the study area, sand content varies from 0.2% to 94.4% with an average of 37.8%, silt content varies from 5.2 to 99.6% with an average of 61.6% and clay content varies from 0 to 2.2% with an average of 0.6% (Fig. 4.3). In overall view, silt is the dominant sediment substrate observed in the estuary which indicates the calm environment due to lack of freshwater influx and confluence of the transient streams

Department of Geology, UNOM

into the estuary. Similar observation was found in Uppanar estuary, where sandy silt is the dominant sediment substrate (Kalpana *et al.,* 2016). A bar mouth (natural pozhi), connects Kappil estuary to the Arabian Sea. But during summertime, unfortunately, a sand bar forms here between estuary and the sea.

### 4.1.4 Kayamkulam

The Pampa and Achankoil rivers empty freshwater through canals into the estuary during flood season. The influence of the ebbing tides of the Arabian Sea into the Kayamkulam estuary is observed almost in all the region. In Kayamkulam the abundance of sand, silt and clay in the sediments of surface sample has been estimated (Table. 4.4). In the study area, sand content varies from 0.4% to 96.6% with an average of 58.10%, silt content varies from 2.2 to 99.4% with an average of 41.5% and clay content varies from 0.2 to 1.2% with an average of 0.4% (Fig. 4.4). Based on the inferences made from the spatial distribution map, sand and silt are the dominant sediment substrate found in the Kayamkulam estuary. Sand proportion is noted higher in the central part of the estuary due to the tidal influx influencing the coarser sediments enters into the estuary. Higher concentration of silt is seen in the northern part of both right and left arm of the estuary indicating the relatively calmer environment due to the lack of confluence of streams or tidal influx. The sediment texture indicates the influence of tidal waters was feeble at the northern and southern margin whereas the central region is highly influenced. Tidal water ebbing winnows finer materials like clay and silt to the sea leaving the coarser sand particles at the region as observed. In southern segment there is a mangrove populated area known as Ayiramthengu where the finer substrate especially silt and sandy silt is dominating due to the organic flocculation and settling of silt from overlying water column. Similar observation was found in Cochin estuary, where sand, sandy silt and silt is dominant sediment substrate (Gandhi *et al.,* 2017).

The determined values are plotted on trilinear diagram. Trefethen's (1950) textural nomenclature has been used to describe the sediment types of the present study area. Taking into consideration the 4 possible sediment types of Trefethen's nomenclature, the substrate of the estuarine sediments, consists of silt, silty sand, sandy silt and sand only (Fig. 4.5 & 4.6). In the sediments of the surface samples from the selected estuaries the relative abundance of the sand, silt and clay at different places shows different composition. Silt, sandy-silt and sand were the main sediment substrate in the selected estuaries (Sajan *et al.,* 1992, Hussain *et al.,* 2020). Silty sediments deposit under calm waters and where the currents are weaker. The coarser sediments were deposited first at the estuarine mouth and the lower reaches of the river due to the density. Whereas at the zone of mixing fine silt dominates as a result of decrease in the flow velocity of the stream and flocculation from intermixing water masses.

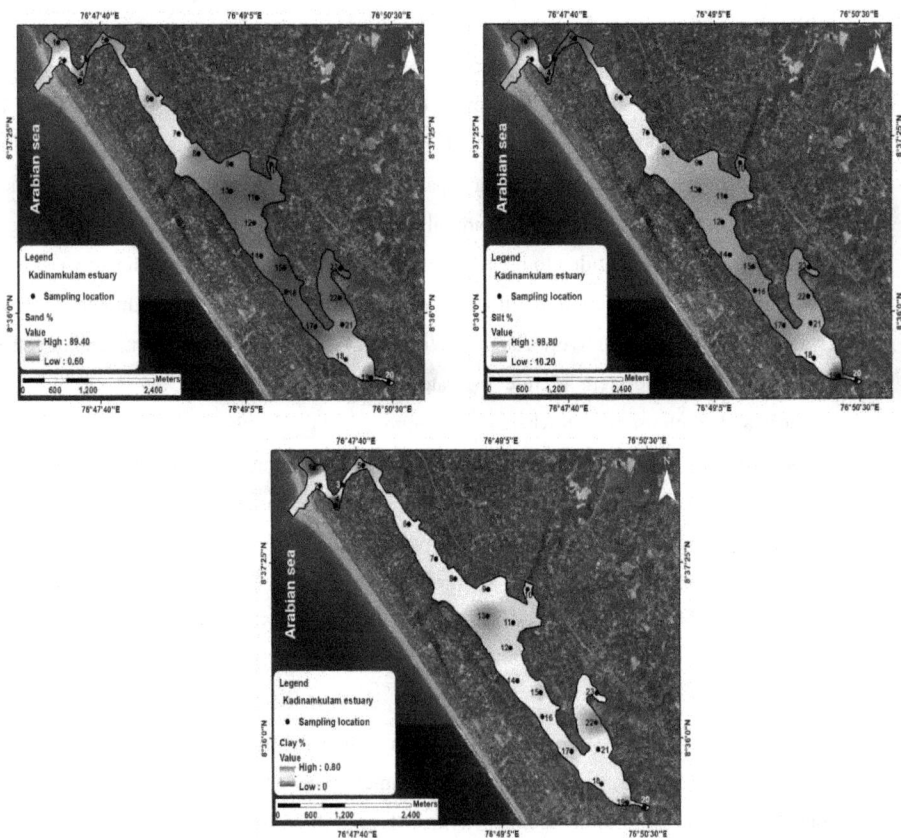

**Fig. 4.1** Representing sediment texture types from surface sediments in Kadinamkulam estuary in Kerala

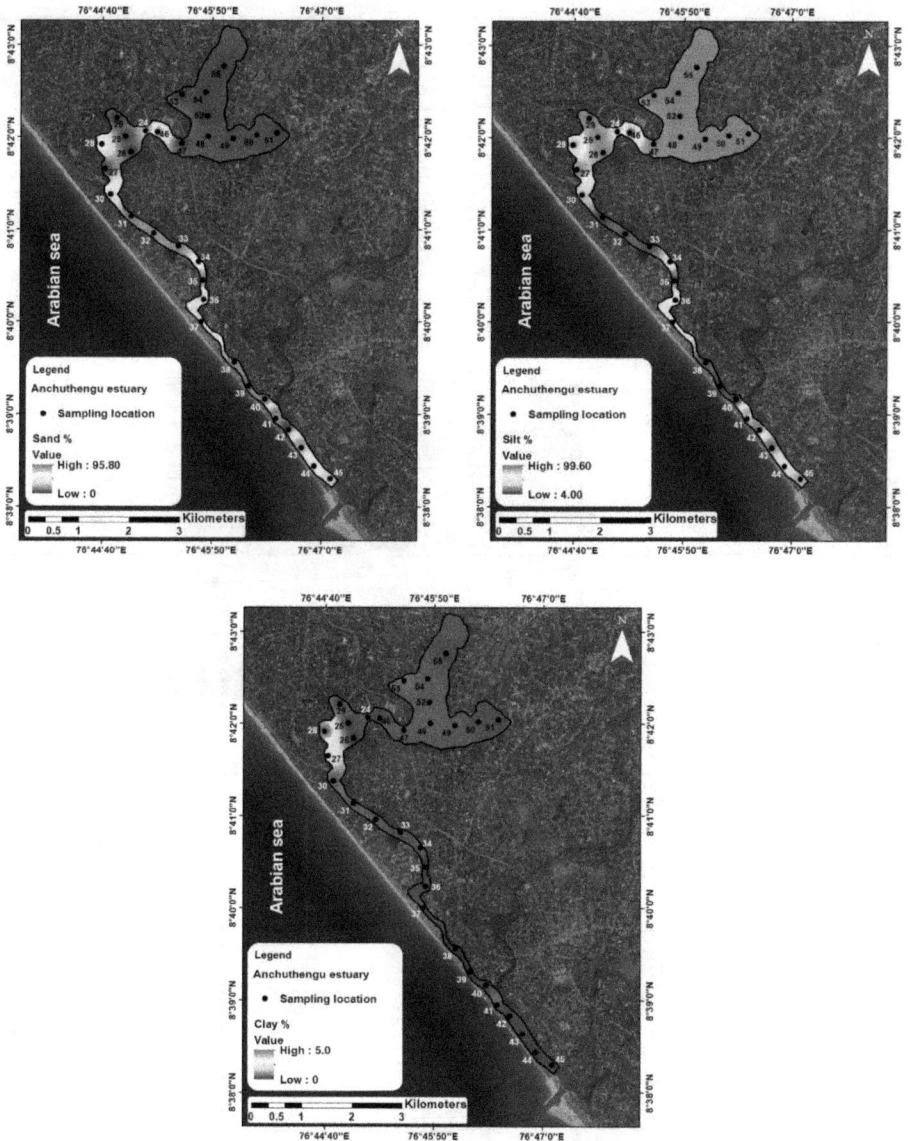

**Fig. 4.2** Representing sediment texture types from surface sediments in Anchuthengu estuary in Kerala

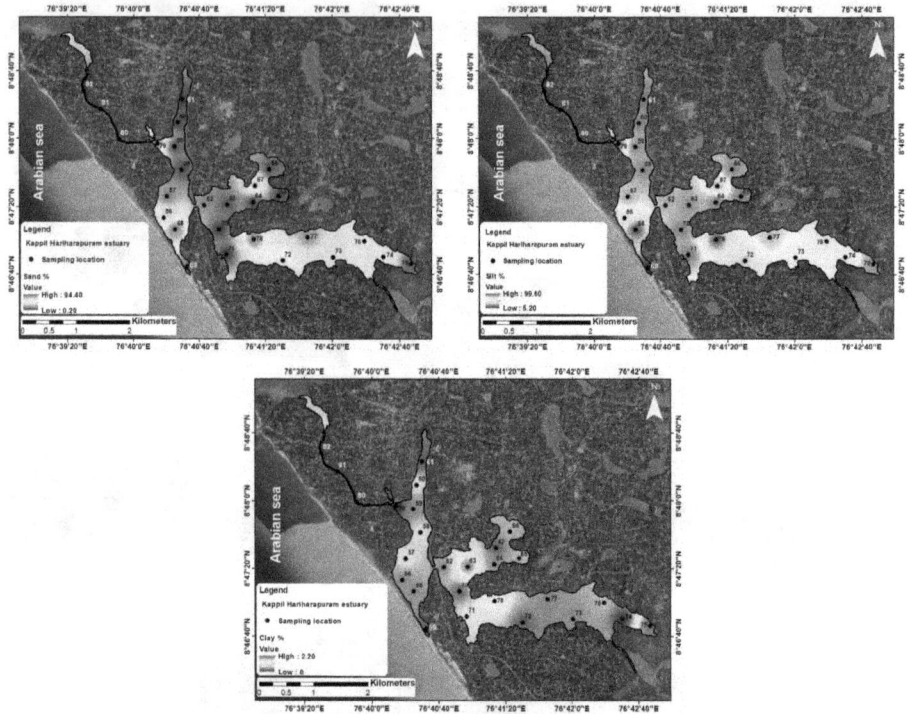

**Fig. 4.3** Representing sediment texture types from surface sediments in Kappil Hariharapuram estuary in Kerala

Department of Geology, UNOM

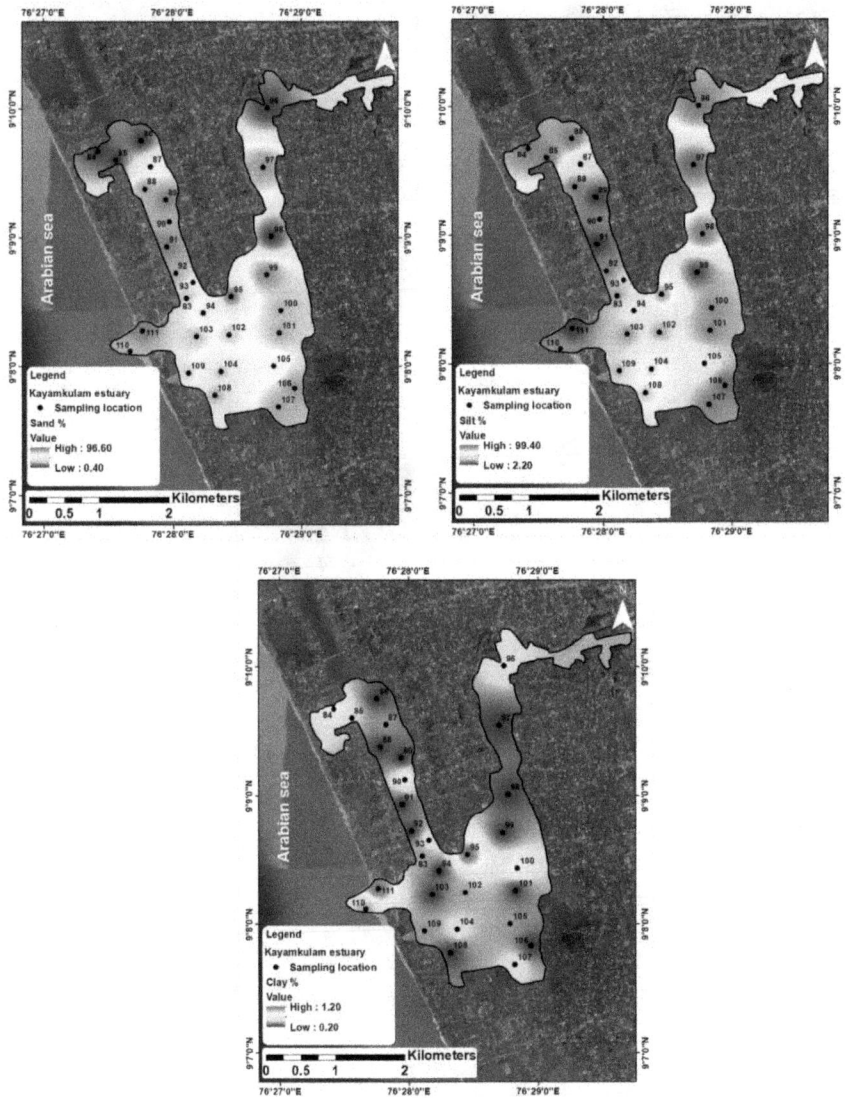

**Fig. 4.4** Representing sediment texture types from surface sediments in Kayamkulam estuary in Kerala

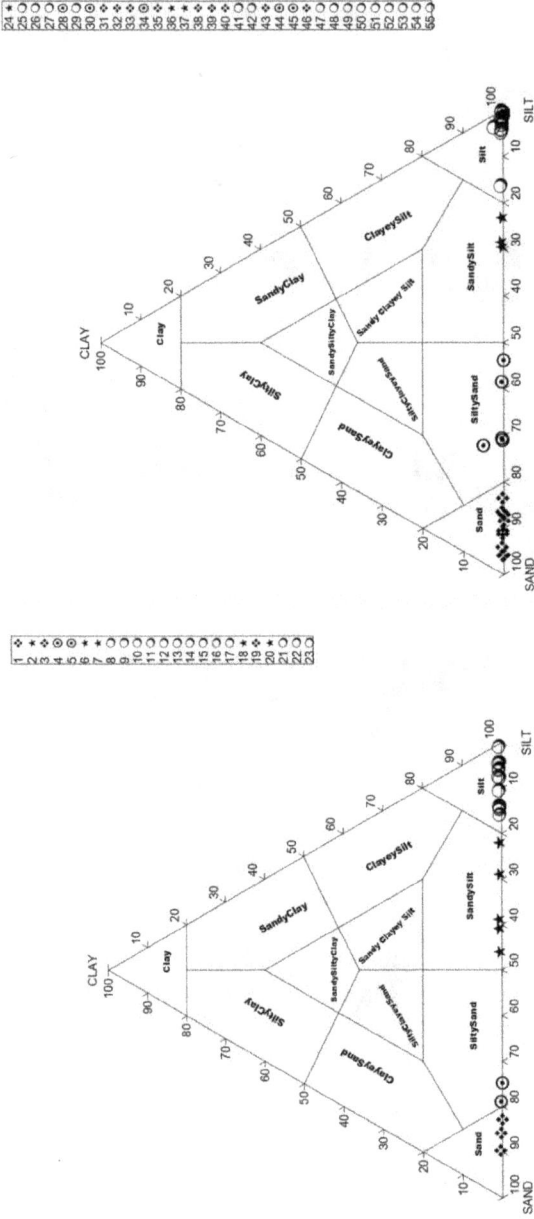

**Fig. 4.5** Trilinear plot on Sand Silt Clay ratio (after Trefethen, 1950) for the surface sediments from Kadinamkulam and Anchuthengu estuary

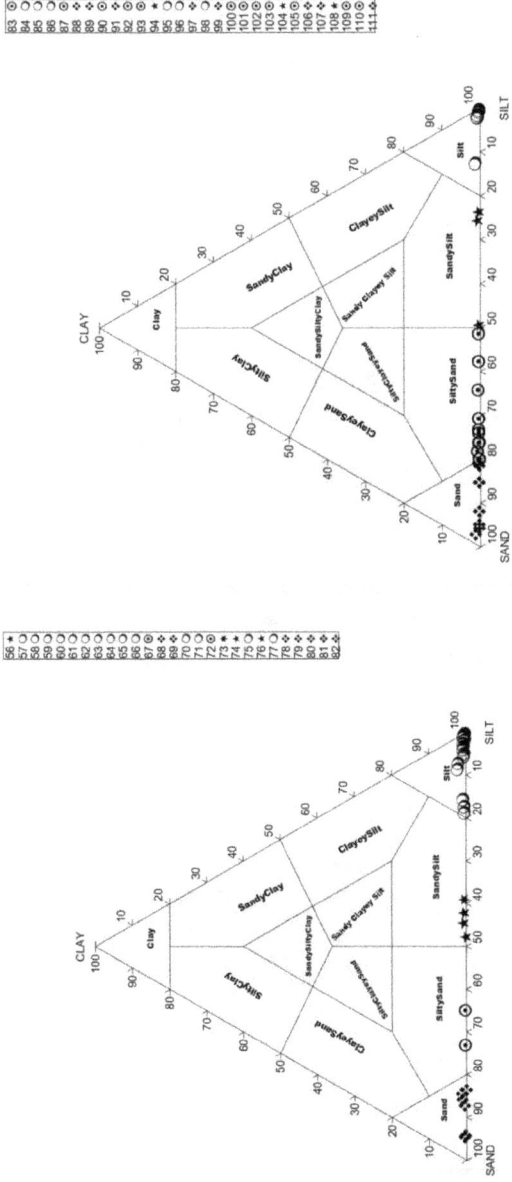

**Fig. 4.6** Trilinear plot on Sand Silt Clay ratio (after Trefethen, 1950) for the surface sediments from Kappil Hariharapuram and Kayamkulam estuary

## 4.2 ORGANIC MATTER

Organic matter is derived from plant forms that thriving on the surface waters of land or on sea. The organic matter in the shallow water region are related with terrigeous plant matertial origin, whereas in the oceans, the source of the organic matter are the photosynthetic planktonic organisms. The organic matter amount depends on rate of depostion of inorganic matter/organic matter, decomposition rate of organic matter or the region's turbluence. Deposition rate of organic matter percentage depends on the upper layer production and destruction rate of bottom water. Excessive oxygen supply cause decomposition of the organic matter at the bottom column. In addition to these factors, sediment texture plays a significant role in preservation of organic matter. Finer grains are less permeable than the coarser grained sediments, where the finer permeable sediments are suitable substrate to preserve the organic matter often. Sverdrup *et al.* (1942) states few conditions that favours higher organic matter content in the sediment formation, the conditions includes good support, relatively faster rate of organic material accumulation and less oxygen supply to the water column contacting the sediment.

Estuaries are the buffer zones controlling wide variety of organic substances, sediments and water from the high efficient terrestrial discharges (Oursel *et al.*, 2013). The estuary act as transitional zone for the multiple contributions from river, sea and land making this pollutants more vulnerable (Kharroubi *et al.*, 2012; Dong *et al.*, 2012; Hu *et al.*, 2013).

### 4.2.1 Kadinamkulam

In the present study, organic matter content was determined for all the surface samples collected (Table. 4.1). The organic matter content in the sediments of surface samples ranges from 0.8 to 8.3 % with an average of 4.7%. The lowest value recorded in station no.5, it's due to abundance of sand and the highest value in station no.17. It is due to abundance of silt and mangrove vegetation (Fig. 4.7). The maximum concentration of OM% is seen in the southern part of the estuary, due to the higher terrigenous materials input and untreated sewage discharge from nearby urbanised regions (Hussain et al., 2020).

Department of Geology, UNOM

### 4.2.2 Anchuthengu

The organic matter content in the sediments of surface samples ranges from 0.9 to 6.8 % with an average of 3.0% (Table. 4.2). The lowest value recorded in station no.42, it's due to abundance of sand and the highest value in station no.29 (Fig. 4.7). The maximum concentration of OM% is seen in the northern part of the estuary its due to the higher terrigenous materials input and untreated sewage discharge from nearby urbanised regions (Hussain *et al.*, 2020).

### 4.2.3 Kappil and Hariharapuram

The organic matter content in the sediments of surface samples ranges from 0.2 to 8.6 % with an average of 3.3% (Table. 4.3). The lowest value recorded in station no.69, it's due to abundance of sand and the highest value in station no.60 (Fig. 4.7). The low OM% in the estuay is due to the constant influence of freshwater (Jonathan *et al.*, 2004).

### 4.2.4 Kayamkulam

The organic matter content in the sediments of surface samples ranges from 0.3 to 13.7 % with an average of 5.9% (Table. 4.4). The lowest value recorded in station no.83, it's due to abundance of sand and the highest value in station no.104 (Fig. 4.7). It is due to abundance of silt and mangrove vegetation. The higher proportion of the organic matter is seen in the southern part of the estuary which lies near Aayiramthengu mangrove a thickly vegetated mangrove area and the right arm of the estuary. Organic content from the magroves might have been influencing the higher values of organic matter in the estuary.

Anthropogenic influences have direct contribution with organic matter inputs from industrial and domestic sewages, agricultural processes, urban runoff and industrial effluents (Mostofa *et al.*, 2012; Watanabe and Kuwae, 2015).

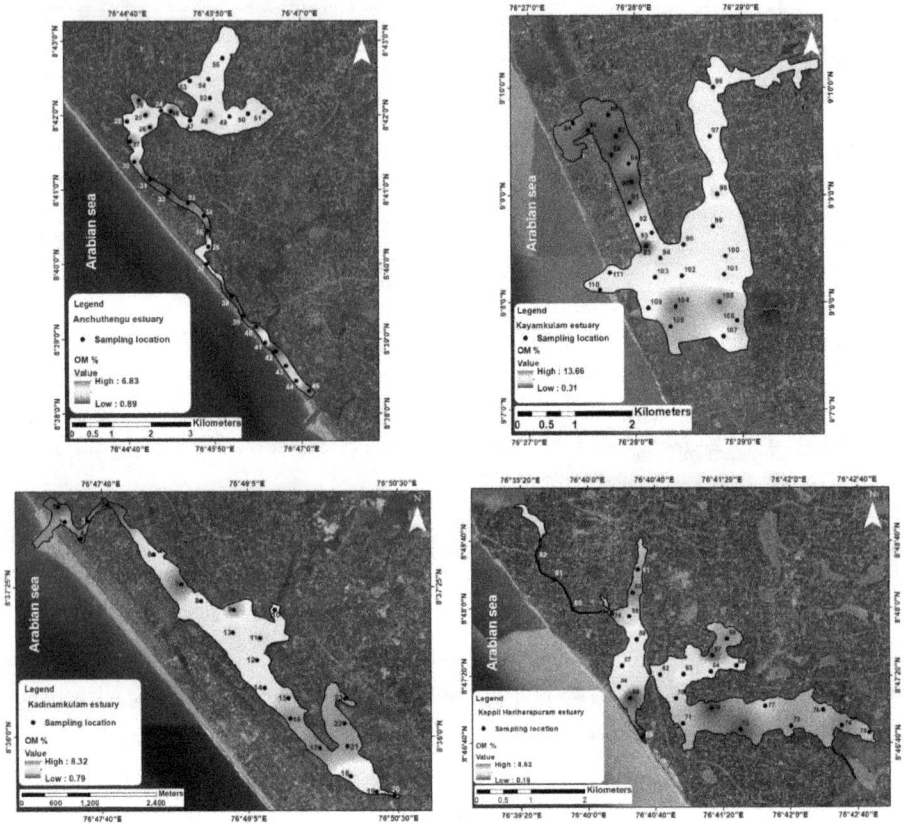

**Fig. 4.7** Representing variations in Organic matter percentages from surface sediments in selective estuaries in Kerala

## 4.3 CALCIUM CARBONATE

The distribution of the calcium carbonate percentages in the surficial sediments was inversely proportional to the organic matter distribution. The higher occurrence of $CaCO_3$ was primarily as a result of calcareous organisms. From the previous published research articles, the above said conclusion was noted on the distribution of $CaCO_3$ and its association with calcareous organisms of the east, west and south coast of India (Jonathan *et al.*, 2004; Kalpana *et al.*, 2016; Saravanan *et al.*, 2018).

### 4.3.1 Kadinamkulam

In the present study, it has been found that the calcium carbonate percentage in the surface sediments in the study area varies from 0.5 to 8.5% with an average of 3.8% (Table. 4.1). The lowest value was recorded in station no. 6 and the highest value in station no.7 (Fig. 4.8) and it is due to the fine-grained materials and absence of shell fragments and also due to the congenial environment for shelled organism respectively. From the observations made on the spatial distribution map shows lower concentrations of CaCO₃ % due to higher concentrations organic matter.

### 4.3.2 Anchuthengu

The calcium carbonate percentage content in the sediments of surface samples ranges from 0.3 to 20.8 % with an average of 4.6% (Table. 4.2). The lowest value recorded in station no.25, is due to abundance of sand and the highest value in station no.37 (Fig. 4.8). It is due to abundance of silty and sandy silt substrate. From the observations made on the spatial distribution map shows lower concentrations of CaCO₃ % due to higher concentrations organic matter.

### 4.3.3 Kappil and Hariharapuram

The calcium carbonate percentage in the sediments of surface samples ranges from 1 to 11.5 % with an average of 5.8% (Table. 4.3). The lowest value recorded in station no.60, is due to abundance of sand and the highest value in station no.82 (Fig. 4.8). It is due to abundance of silty substrates. Elevated percentages of calcium carboante content reported at the estuary is due to the leaching of shelled organisms. Similar finding were also reported by Santhosh (2002) at Paravur- Kappil backwater.

### 4.3.4 Kayamkulam

The calcium carbonate percentage in the sediments of surface samples ranges from 0.5 to 21.5 % with an average of 4.5% (Table. 4.4). The lowest value recorded in station no.109, is due to abundance of sand and the highest value in station no.104 (Fig. 4.8). It is due to abundance of silt and mangrove remains.

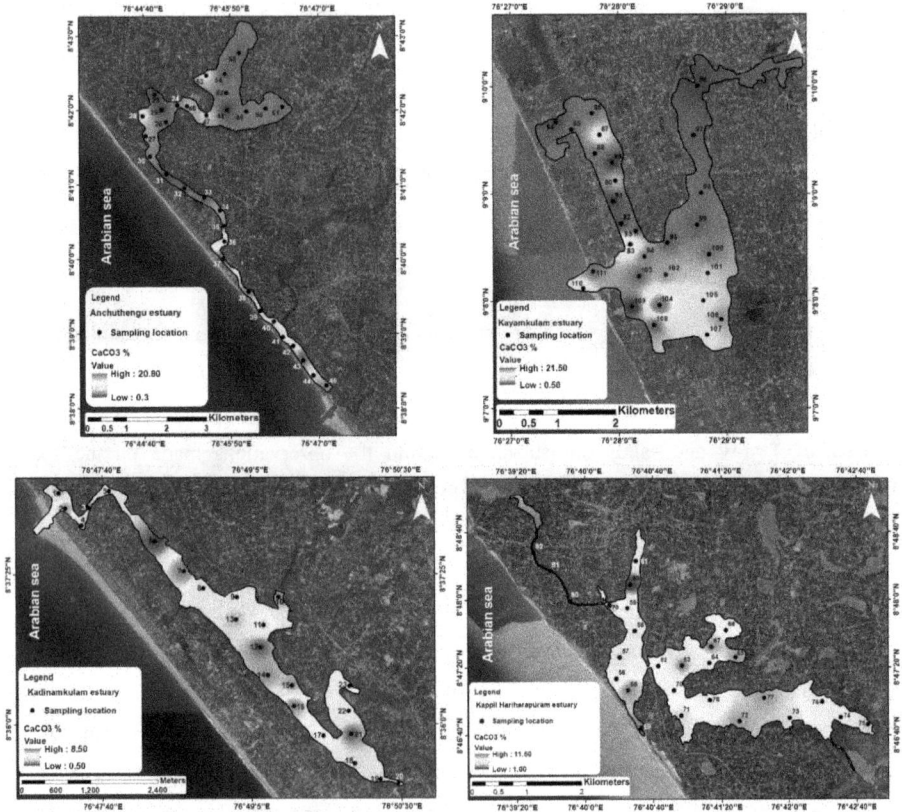

**Fig. 4.8** Representing variations in CaCO$_3$ percentages from surface sediments in selective estuaries in Kerala

Department of Geology, UNOM

**Table. 4.1** Sediment texture, CaCO₃ and Organic Matter (in percentage) in surface sediments of the
Kadinamkulam estuary, Kerala

| Sample No | Sand | Silt | Clay | OM | CaCO₃ | Sediment substrate |
|---|---|---|---|---|---|---|
| 1 | 82.8 | 17.2 | 0.0 | 1.2 | 2.5 | Sand |
| 2 | 40.6 | 58.8 | 0.6 | 3.0 | 7.5 | Sandy silt |
| 3 | 89.4 | 10.2 | 0.4 | 2.5 | 2.5 | Sand |
| 4 | 74.8 | 25.2 | 0.0 | 2.0 | 4.0 | Silty sand |
| 5 | 78.8 | 21.0 | 0.2 | 0.8 | 4.5 | Silty sand |
| 6 | 21.8 | 77.8 | 0.4 | 4.7 | 0.5 | Sandy silt |
| 7 | 45.8 | 53.8 | 0.4 | 1.6 | 8.5 | Sandy silt |
| 8 | 14.0 | 85.6 | 0.4 | 4.1 | 3.5 | Silt |
| 9 | 13.8 | 85.8 | 0.4 | 7.6 | 3.5 | Silt |
| 10 | 10.2 | 89.2 | 0.6 | 3.6 | 2.0 | Silt |
| 11 | 5.4 | 94.0 | 0.6 | 3.1 | 6.5 | Silt |
| 12 | 13.6 | 85.8 | 0.6 | 5.0 | 1.0 | Silt |
| 13 | 7.0 | 92.2 | 0.8 | 3.8 | 2.5 | Silt |
| 14 | 14.4 | 85.2 | 0.4 | 5.0 | 2.0 | Silt |
| 15 | 0.6 | 98.8 | 0.6 | 6.5 | 2.0 | Silt |
| 16 | 4.2 | 95.4 | 0.4 | 7.6 | 8.0 | Silt |
| 17 | 5.6 | 93.8 | 0.6 | 8.3 | 6.0 | Silt |
| 18 | 28.8 | 70.8 | 0.4 | 4.5 | 3.0 | Sandy silt |
| 19 | 85.8 | 14.0 | 0.2 | 3.3 | 3.0 | Sand |
| 20 | 38.6 | 60.8 | 0.6 | 7.4 | 3.5 | Sandy silt |
| 21 | 15.6 | 84.0 | 0.4 | 7.8 | 1.0 | Silt |
| 22 | 4.0 | 95.2 | 0.8 | 7.8 | 4.5 | Silt |
| 23 | 7.4 | 92.2 | 0.4 | 7.4 | 5.5 | Silt |
| Avg | 30.6 | 69.0 | 0.4 | 4.7 | 3.8 | |
| Max | 89.4 | 98.8 | 0.8 | 8.3 | 8.5 | |
| Min | 0.6 | 10.2 | 0.0 | 0.8 | 0.5 | |

**Table. 4.2** Sediment texture, CaCO₃ and Organic Matter (in percentage) in surface sediments of the Anchuthengu estuary, Kerala

| Sample No | Sand | Silt | Clay | OM | CaCO₃ | Sediment substrate |
|:---:|:---:|:---:|:---:|:---:|:---:|:---:|
| 24 | 23.0 | 76.8 | 0.2 | 3.5 | 3.3 | Sandy silt |
| 25 | 1.4 | 98.6 | 0.0 | 1.8 | 0.3 | Silt |
| 26 | 0.6 | 99.4 | 0.0 | 5.8 | 2.3 | Silt |
| 27 | 2.6 | 95.2 | 2.2 | 6.5 | 4.3 | Silt |
| 28 | 69.6 | 25.4 | 5.0 | 3.0 | 7.5 | Silty sand |
| 29 | 0.2 | 99.6 | 0.2 | 6.8 | 0.8 | Silt |
| 30 | 70.4 | 29.2 | 0.4 | 2.3 | 3.3 | Silty sand |
| 31 | 93.8 | 5.8 | 0.4 | 1.1 | 1.3 | Sand |
| 32 | 86.2 | 13.4 | 0.4 | 1.2 | 2.0 | Sand |
| 33 | 91.2 | 8.6 | 0.2 | 1.6 | 2.3 | Sand |
| 34 | 58.2 | 41.4 | 0.4 | 2.1 | 4.3 | Silty sand |
| 35 | 88.4 | 11.6 | 0.0 | 1.2 | 3.3 | Sand |
| 36 | 29.4 | 70.4 | 0.2 | 4.4 | 8.0 | Sandy silt |
| 37 | 28.2 | 71.4 | 0.4 | 4.3 | 20.8 | Sandy silt |
| 38 | 87.0 | 13.0 | 0.0 | 1.0 | 3.8 | Sand |
| 39 | 95.8 | 4.2 | 0.0 | 1.3 | 8.3 | Sand |
| 40 | 95.8 | 4.0 | 0.2 | 1.4 | 7.3 | Sand |
| 41 | 16.0 | 83.4 | 0.6 | 4.5 | 9.3 | Silt |
| 42 | 3.0 | 96.8 | 0.2 | 0.9 | 9.3 | Silt |
| 43 | 83.4 | 16.4 | 0.2 | 2.5 | 2.0 | Sand |
| 44 | 53.8 | 46.2 | 0.0 | 3.4 | 6.3 | Silty sand |
| 45 | 71.0 | 28.8 | 0.2 | 1.8 | 3.8 | Silty sand |
| 46 | 90.4 | 9.4 | 0.2 | 1.3 | 5.5 | Sand |
| 47 | 1.8 | 97.8 | 0.4 | 3.7 | 6.0 | Silt |
| 48 | 4.6 | 95.0 | 0.4 | 2.0 | 0.5 | Silt |
| 49 | 4.0 | 95.6 | 0.4 | 5.0 | 3.0 | Silt |
| 50 | 4.0 | 95.8 | 0.2 | 3.6 | 3.0 | Silt |
| 51 | 2.4 | 97.4 | 0.2 | 2.9 | 2.5 | Silt |
| 52 | 0.0 | 99.6 | 0.4 | 3.9 | 2.5 | Silt |
| 53 | 1.4 | 98.0 | 0.6 | 3.5 | 6.5 | Silt |
| 54 | 2.0 | 97.6 | 0.4 | 3.4 | 1.5 | Silt |
| 55 | 1.6 | 98.2 | 0.2 | 4.4 | 2.0 | Silt |
| **Avg** | **39.4** | **60.1** | **0.5** | **3.0** | **4.6** | |
| **Max** | **95.8** | **99.6** | **5.0** | **6.8** | **20.8** | |
| **Min** | **0.0** | **4.0** | **0.0** | **0.9** | **0.3** | |

**Table. 4.3** Sediment texture, CaCO₃ and Organic Matter (in percentage) in surface sediments of the Kappil- Hariharapuram estuary, Kerala

| Sample No | Sand | Silt | Clay | OM | CaCO₃ | Sediment substrate |
|-----------|------|------|------|-----|-------|--------------------|
| 56 | 42.0 | 57.6 | 0.4 | 4.5 | 5.0 | Sandy silt |
| 57 | 15.2 | 84.0 | 0.8 | 5.7 | 3.5 | Silt |
| 58 | 3.6 | 95.6 | 0.8 | 4.4 | 4.0 | Silt |
| 59 | 4.8 | 94.8 | 0.4 | 6.2 | 6.5 | Silt |
| 60 | 2.2 | 97.0 | 0.8 | 8.6 | 1.0 | Silt |
| 61 | 0.2 | 99.6 | 0.2 | 7.2 | 5.0 | Silt |
| 62 | 17.2 | 82.4 | 0.4 | 3.5 | 6.0 | Silt |
| 63 | 6.2 | 91.8 | 2.0 | 5.5 | 2.5 | Silt |
| 64 | 0.8 | 98.8 | 0.4 | 5.2 | 4.0 | Silt |
| 65 | 3.0 | 96.4 | 0.6 | 3.4 | 7.5 | Silt |
| 66 | 5.4 | 94.0 | 0.6 | 1.9 | 5.5 | Silt |
| 67 | 73.0 | 26.8 | 0.2 | 0.7 | 8.0 | Silty sand |
| 68 | 87.0 | 12.6 | 0.4 | 0.4 | 8.0 | Sand |
| 69 | 94.0 | 5.8 | 0.2 | 0.2 | 8.3 | Sand |
| 70 | 1.6 | 98.2 | 0.2 | 2.9 | 5.5 | Silt |
| 71 | 0.4 | 98.8 | 0.8 | 2.6 | 6.5 | Silt |
| 72 | 64.8 | 35.0 | 0.2 | 0.8 | 7.5 | Silty sand |
| 73 | 39.0 | 60.6 | 0.4 | 2.0 | 6.5 | Sandy silt |
| 74 | 47.8 | 52.2 | 0.0 | 1.8 | 5.5 | Sandy silt |
| 75 | 7.6 | 90.2 | 2.2 | 2.6 | 3.5 | Silt |
| 76 | 44.4 | 55.0 | 0.6 | 2.4 | 5.0 | Sandy silt |
| 77 | 18.6 | 81.0 | 0.4 | 3.0 | 7.5 | Silt |
| 78 | 83.8 | 15.0 | 1.2 | 0.5 | 5.0 | Sand |
| 79 | 83.6 | 16.4 | 0.0 | 8.3 | 7.0 | Sand |
| 80 | 94.2 | 5.6 | 0.2 | 0.9 | 5.0 | Sand |
| 81 | 94.4 | 5.2 | 0.4 | 2.2 | 5.0 | Sand |
| 82 | 85.4 | 13.6 | 1.0 | 1.9 | 11.5 | Sand |
| **Avg** | **37.8** | **61.6** | **0.6** | **3.3** | **5.8** | |
| **Max** | **94.4** | **99.6** | **2.2** | **8.6** | **11.5** | |
| **Min** | **0.2** | **5.2** | **0.0** | **0.2** | **1.0** | |

**Table. 4.4** Sediment texture, CaCO₃ and Organic Matter (in percentage) in surface sediments of the Kayamkulam estuary, Kerala

| Sample No | Sand | Silt | Clay | OM | CaCO$_3$ | Sediment substrate |
|:---:|:---:|:---:|:---:|:---:|:---:|:---:|
| 83 | 73.0 | 26.6 | 0.4 | 0.3 | 14.5 | Silty sand |
| 84 | 1.6 | 97.6 | 0.8 | 2.4 | 1.5 | Silt |
| 85 | 1.4 | 98.1 | 0.5 | 0.5 | 3.0 | Silt |
| 86 | 0.4 | 99.4 | 0.2 | 1.6 | 3.0 | Silt |
| 87 | 57.6 | 42.0 | 0.4 | 0.4 | 8.5 | Silty sand |
| 88 | 81.4 | 18.4 | 0.2 | 0.6 | 3.0 | Sand |
| 89 | 94.8 | 5.0 | 0.2 | 3.0 | 1.0 | Sand |
| 90 | 77.8 | 21.4 | 0.8 | 0.5 | 5.5 | Silty sand |
| 91 | 95.6 | 4.2 | 0.2 | 1.1 | 1.5 | Sand |
| 92 | 79.8 | 20.0 | 0.2 | 8.7 | 1.5 | Silty sand |
| 93 | 64.0 | 35.4 | 0.6 | 8.9 | 2.5 | Silty sand |
| 94 | 49.4 | 50.4 | 0.2 | 4.7 | 3.5 | Sandy silt |
| 95 | 12.0 | 86.8 | 1.2 | 4.3 | 2.5 | Silt |
| 96 | 1.8 | 97.6 | 0.6 | 8.9 | 1.5 | Silt |
| 97 | 85.2 | 14.6 | 0.2 | 7.8 | 2.5 | Sand |
| 98 | 0.8 | 99.0 | 0.2 | 9.3 | 3.0 | Silt |
| 99 | 91.8 | 8.0 | 0.2 | 5.5 | 2.5 | Sand |
| 100 | 77.8 | 21.4 | 0.8 | 5.9 | 3.0 | Silty sand |
| 101 | 79.8 | 20.0 | 0.2 | 6.2 | 6.0 | Silty sand |
| 102 | 73.8 | 25.8 | 0.4 | 8.4 | 4.5 | Silty sand |
| 103 | 76.0 | 23.8 | 0.2 | 8.4 | 2.5 | Silty sand |
| 104 | 25.4 | 74.0 | 0.6 | 13.7 | 21.5 | Sandy silt |
| 105 | 51.2 | 48.4 | 0.4 | 12.0 | 7.5 | Silty sand |
| 106 | 85.2 | 14.6 | 0.2 | 10.1 | 4.5 | Sand |
| 107 | 80.6 | 18.8 | 0.6 | 8.0 | 7.0 | Sand |
| 108 | 23.6 | 76.2 | 0.2 | 10.9 | 2.5 | Sandy silt |
| 109 | 70.6 | 29.0 | 0.4 | 7.6 | 0.5 | Silty sand |
| 110 | 76.0 | 23.6 | 0.4 | 4.9 | 8.0 | Silty sand |
| 111 | 96.6 | 2.2 | 1.2 | 7.2 | 3.0 | Sand |
| **Avg** | **58.1** | **41.5** | **0.4** | **5.9** | **4.5** | |
| **Max** | **96.6** | **99.4** | **1.2** | **13.7** | **21.5** | |
| **Min** | **0.4** | **2.2** | **0.2** | **0.3** | **0.5** | |

Department of Geology, UNOM

# CHAPTER - V

# ELEMENTAL CONCENTRATION AND POLLUTION INDICES

## 5.1 INTRODUCTION

Sediments have the ability to carry the elements and could behave as a sink for various contaminants in aquatic environments, particularly in marginal marine environment (Wang *et al.,* 2014; Liu *et al.,* 2019; Herbert *et al.,* 2020). The estuarine and marine biota have a negative impact from the toxic elements existing in the aquatic environment (Nagarajan *et al.,* 2014; Islam *et al.,* 2017). Physical, chemical and biological processes control the elemental concentration distribution in sediments (Ramanathan *et al.,* 1999; Selvam *et al.,* 2012). Even lower levels of toxic elements available to biological cycle are very harmful. There is a great need to understand the behavior of the trace elements distribution to encounter the problems in organisms by pollution (Negri and Heyward, 2001). Cearreta *et al. (*2000) states that the major source of pollutants along the marginal marine and marine environment was anthropogenic factors followed by natural weathering. Estuarine sediments were discovered to be the main entry point for pollutants into the open sea. Riverine metals generated from geogenic and manmade sources are filtered by estuaries (Larrose *et al.,* 2010). Due to its abundance, persistence and environmental toxicity, trace element contamination in the estuaries attain global attention (Ali *et al.,* 2016; Hwang *et al.,* 2016).

In order to study the problem of metal contamination in coastal and estuarine environments, rigorous investigations have been carried out to address its effects on biota and sediment profiles (Liu *et al.,* 2016; Jonathan *et al.,* 2016; Baran *et al.,* 2019). At the end of nineteenth century industrial revolution in Indian subcontinent markup the beginning of enrichment of trace metals in sediment profiles. In the aquatic environments trace metals ultimately sink in the sediments (Caccia *et al.,* 2003). Hence the history of the weathering pattern and metal accumulation of the sediments from nearby regions was reflected by the solid phase distribution in the sediments (Forstner and Salomons 1980; Nath *et al.,* 2000). The extensively studied trace elements in the last decade were Cu, Pb, Zn, Ni, Co, Cr, Cd, As, Fe, Mn, Se and B (He *et al.,* 2005). Some of these elements were essential to the metabolic growth of plants (Cu, Fe, Mn, Zn, B and Mo), some elements like Cd and Pb were worrisome to the environment contaminating the water, soil and food chains (Islam *et al.,* 2018). Geogenic elements such as Fe, Zn and Cu becomes toxic at higher concentrations, whereas elements including Cd, Pb and As are capable of being mutagenic, carcinogenic or teratogenic materials (Yoshida *et al.,* 2006).

A vast spectrum of pollution indices was used to evaluate trace element-based ecological risk and environmental issues in the estuaries. Polluted indices are an important instrument for assessing, processing, and communicating environmental data to the general public, specialists, and lawmakers (Caeiro *et al.,* 2005). The Enrichment Factor (EF), Contamination Factor (CF), Geo-accumulation Index ($I_{geo}$), Potential Ecological Risk Index (PERI) are some pollution indices mostly used in dealing the environmental issues. For studying the pollution indices calculations, the lowest value of the local background concentration (Jeshma, 2020; unpublished thesis) was used from three core samples (Length of the cores = C1 - 0.56 m, C2 - 0 .68 m, & C3 - 1.04 m) (Table 5.1).

## 5.2 DISTRIBUTION OF IRON, MANGANESE AND TRACE ELEMENTS IN THE SURFACE SEDIMENT

### 5.2.1 Iron (Fe)

Iron has two oxidation states Fe $2^+$ and Fe $3^+$ is the fourth abundant element and also vital element for plants and humans (Riley and Chester, 1971; Anbuselvan and Sridharan, 2018). The concentration of iron (Fe) in the Kadinamkulam estuary ranges from 7681.37 to 31438.17 ppm with an average 19893.76 ppm (Table. 5.1). The maximum and minimum concentration of Fe was noticed in sample number 17 and 2, respectively and shown in the map (Fig. 5.1). The distribution of Fe at the Anchuthengu estuary ranges from 12914.99 to 158639.33 ppm with an average of 30842.49 ppm. The maximum and minimum values were found at sample numbers 44 and 32, respectively (Table. 5.2). The concentration of Fe varies from 14204.11 to 47533.91 ppm with a mean value of 26037.33ppm in the Kappil- Hariharapuram estuary. The higher and lower concentrations observed in the sampling locations 63 and 68 (Table. 5.3). The distribution of iron concentration ranges from 8086.75 to 42163.35 ppm with the average of 23565.98 ppm noted in the Kayamkulam estuary. The higher and lower concentrations of Fe were noted in the sampling locations 101 and 92, respectively (Table. 5.4). The concentration of iron observed in the study area was lower than the local background value (Jeshma, 2020) and the upper continental crust

Department of Geology, UNOM

(UCC) value. The inflow of the riverine sediments enriches the iron concentration in these estuaries which was supported by the spatial map of iron (Fig. 5.1). The weathering and deposition of the surficial sediments during the monsoonal showers along the estuarine banks contributes the iron concentrations into the estuarine sediments.

### 5.2.2 Manganese (Mn)

The mean concentration of manganese in various geologic sources like ultramafic, mafic granitic, basaltic, shale, limestone and sandstone rocks were 1040 ppm, 1500 ppm, 390 ppm, 1500 ppm, 850 ppm, 620 ppm and 460 ppm, respectively (Bowen, 1979). In industrial sources and natural weathering products manganese exists as manganese oxides. The Manganese concentration in Kadinamkulam estuary ranges from 91.95 to 887.59 ppm and its average value are 242.91 ppm (Table. 5.1). The higher concentration of Mn value at the Station no 3, and lowest value at the Station no 2 are recorded. The concentration of Mn fluctuates from 68.19 to 1063.84 ppm with a mean value of 279.61 ppm in the Anchuthengu estuary. The higher and lower concentrations observed in the sampling locations 48 and 37 (Table. 5.2). The distribution of Mn at the Kappil-Hariharapuram estuary ranges from 146.37 to 768.58 ppm with an average of 292.69 ppm. The maximum and minimum values were found at sample numbers 62 and 80 respectively (Table. 5.3). The concentration of Mn in the Kayamkulam estuary ranges from 178.94 to 443.27 ppm with an average 316.81 ppm (Table. 5.1). The maximum and minimum concentration of Mn was noticed in sample number 84 and 92, respectively and represented in the figure (Fig. 5.2).

Lower concentrations of Mn at the surficial sediments denotes that dissolved Mn ions with higher mobility are readily removed from the pore water of sediments to the water column through advection and diffusion processes (Janaki- Raman *et al.,* 2007). The deposition of the trace elements in the estuarine sediments was aided by the hydrodynamics, frequently caused by interaction with salinity, pH, temperature and redox effects (Jayaprakash *et al.,* 2014). The concentration of Mn observed in the study area was lower than the upper continental crust (UCC) value.

### 5.2.3 Lead (Pb)

Lead of inorganic origin is toxic to aquatic plants and to invertebrates' similar mercury, copper, zinc and cadmium. Alkyl-lead an organic compound often used as antiknock agents in petroleum products is toxic to life forms (Denton *et al.,* 1997). The Lead concentration in Kadinamkulam estuary ranges from 42.05 to 94.23 ppm and its average value are 76.48 ppm (Table. 5.1). The higher concentration of Pb value at the Station no 22, and lowest value at the Station no 3 are recorded. The concentration of Pb varies from 38.70 to 116.55 ppm with a mean value of 73.55 ppm in the Anchuthengu estuary. The higher and lower concentrations observed in the sampling locations 55 and 31, respectively (Table. 5.2). The distribution of Pb at the Kappil-Hariharapuram estuary ranges from 73.34 to 108.10 ppm with an average of 95.91 ppm. The maximum and minimum values were found at sample numbers 59 and 76, respectively (Table. 5.3). The concentration of Pb in the Kayamkulam estuary ranges from 82.4 to 107.68 ppm with an average 92.33 ppm (Table. 5.4). The maximum and minimum concentration of Pb was noticed in sample number 85 and 105, respectively and shown (Fig. 5.3). Untreated urban discharges and sewages were the reasons for higher concentration of Pb. The dominance of silt and organic matter allows absorption of Pb from the water column (Robin *et al.,* 2012). Probable origin of Pb is derived from the effluents of industries and domestic sewages or through engine fuel spills of boats (El Sayed and Basaham, 2004; Abu-Zied *et al.,* 2013).

### 5.2.4 Zinc (Zn)

Abundance of detrital oxides, ferromagnesian silicates control the dispersion of zinc in sediments (Wedepohl *et al.,* 1978). Zinc's mobility in the environment is active acidic, oxidizing conditions whereas restricted in reduced conditions. Various industrial activities are the main anthropogenic sources of zinc, one such is using of zinc as coating against corrosion. Zn production is increasing globally due to its industrial uses which lead to the dispersal of the metal widely in the environment. As a result, the Zn concentration increased higher than pre-industrial level in various segment of the environment.

The concentration of zinc in the Kadinamkulam estuary ranges from 13.70 to 224.03 ppm with an average 130.96 ppm (Table. 5.1). The maximum and minimum concentration of Zn was noticed in sample number 4 and 3, respectively and is shown (Fig. 5.4). The distribution of Zn at the Anchuthengu estuary ranges from 62.20 to 237.03 ppm with an average of 122.58 ppm. The maximum and minimum values were found at sample numbers 49 and 28, respectively (Table. 5.2). The concentration of Zn varies from 65.60 to 369.61 ppm with a mean value of 192.07 ppm in the Kappil- Hariharapuram estuary. The higher and lower concentrations observed in the sampling locations 67 and 80, respectively (Table. 5.3). The distribution of Zn concentration ranges from 55.93 to 198.78 ppm with the average of 107.75 ppm noted in the Kayamkulam estuary. The higher and lower concentrations were noted in the sampling locations 83 and 92 respectively (Table. 5.4). The concentration of Zn observed in the study area was higher than the upper continental crust (UCC) value and local background value. River runoff is the major source for zinc from industrial sources including wastewater, fishing, foundries, etc., and domestic sewages.

### 5.2.5 Copper (Cu)

Copper is a commonly found element in nature and also used by humans from the earlier stages of their civilization. It is an essential element for all life forms since it is used in their metabolic cycle. Distribution of Cu is aided with scavenging and local inputs along with involvement in biological cycle (Nolting *et al.*, 1991). The concentration of Cu in the Kadinamkulam estuary ranges from 5.97 to 163.95 ppm with an average 66.57 ppm (Table. 5.1). The maximum and minimum concentration of Cu was noticed in sample number 1 and 3, respectively and is represented in the figure (Fig. 5.5). The distribution of Cu at the Anchuthengu estuary ranges from 16.91 to 182.97 ppm with an average of 71.23 ppm. The maximum and minimum values were found at sample numbers 26 and 32 respectively (Table. 5.2). The concentration of Cu varies from 35.30 to 607.29 ppm with a mean value of 143.74 ppm in the Kappil- Hariharapuram estuary. The higher and lower concentrations observed in the sampling locations 69 and 64 (Table. 5.3). The distribution of Cu concentration ranges from 9.91 to 52.62 ppm with the average of 25.07 ppm noted in the Kayamkulam estuary. The higher and lower concentrations were noted in the sampling locations 94 and 102 respectively (Table. 5.4). The concentration of copper in the estuarine sediments implicates that it is derived from the fluvial and natural weathering processes. The concentration of Cu observed in the study area was higher than the upper continental crust (UCC) value. In the sediment substrate the decomposed leaves accumulate higher percentage of Cu and also attribution from antifoulants used in boats.

Department of Geology, UNOM

### 5.2.6 Chromium (Cr)

The natural weathering processes bring chromium into the estuarine system. Chromium species availability in the sediments was reduced in pore water post precipitation or by microbial action during carbonate precipitation (Fang *et al.*, 2021). Anthropogenic factors including the confluence of sewage and wastewater from textile, leather and steel manufacturing plants into the environment which results in the increasing concentration of chromium in the environment. The Cr concentration in Kadinamkulam estuary ranges from 11.91 to 396.18 ppm and its average value are 251.61 ppm (Table. 5.1). The concentration of Cr varies from 172.46 to 540.21 ppm with a mean value of 272.58 ppm in the Anchuthengu estuary (Table. 5.2). Whereas the distribution of Cr at the Kappil- Hariharapuram estuary ranges from 203.30 to 378.29 ppm with an average of 283.84 ppm (Table. 5.3). The concentration of Cr in the Kayamkulam estuary ranges from 206.19 to 764.33 ppm with an average 331.77 ppm (Table. 5.4). Comparing to other three estuaries the mean concentration of Cr is relatively higher in Kayamkulam estuary, this may be due to the sand-rich sediment substrate seen at the estuarine mouth (Fig. 5.6). The concentration of Cr observed in the study area was higher than the upper continental crust (UCC) value and local background value. Distribution of non-detrital elements like Cr depends upon the Mn- oxides and Al-rich finer fractions (Selvaraj *et al.*, 2004). The primary sources for the higher concentration of chromium in the estuarine sediments are human caused sources like sewage and runoff from urban zones (Gopal *et al.*, 2018).

### 5.2.7 Nickel (Ni)

Nickel has wide range of applications such as metallurgical alloy, electroplating, in batteries and as catalyst. Ni reaches the landfills through sewage containing battery and metal plate wastes. With prevailing anaerobic condition in estuarine bottom sediments, mobility of nickel was tending to be controlled by sulfide. But the major factor controlling the Ni in these conditions were nickeliferous iron oxides or nickel hydroxides (Callender, 2005). Nickel compounds have the tendency to be a carcinogen to humans and also when exposed frequently affects lung functioning (Finkelman, 2005).

The concentration of Ni in the Kadinamkulam estuary ranges from 19.87 to 163.75 ppm with an average 112.30 ppm (Table. 5.1). the higher and lower concentration is observed at sample no. 23 and sample no. 3, respectively and the same is shown in figure (Fig. 5.7). The distribution of Ni at the Anchuthengu estuary ranges from 72.80 to 338.68 ppm with an average of 119.73 ppm. The maximum and minimum values were found at sample numbers 28 and 31, respectively (Table. 5.2). The concentration of Ni varies from 92.33 to 180.67 ppm with a mean value of 127.36 ppm in the Kappil- Hariharapuram estuary (Table. 5.3). The distribution of Ni concentration ranges from 88.75 to 450.98 ppm (Table 5.4) with the average of 135.11 ppm noted in the Kayamkulam estuary. The higher and lower concentrations were noted in the sampling locations 96 and 92, respectively. The concentration of Ni observed in the study area was higher than the upper continental crust (UCC) value. The Ni concentration shows association with anthropogenic sources (Ma and Hooda, 2010; Gopal *et al.*, 2018 and Hussain *et al.*, 2020).

### 5.2.8 Cobalt (Co)

The concentration of Co in the Kadinamkulam estuary ranges from 1.04 to 41.26 ppm with an average 33.02 ppm (Table. 5.1) and at the Anchuthengu estuary ranges from 27.73 to 48.22 ppm with an average of 39.04 ppm (Table. 5.2). It varies from 12.50 to 44.85 ppm with a mean value of 35.17 ppm in the Kappil- Hariharapuram estuary (Table. 5.3). The distribution of Ni concentration ranges from 19.28 to 152.13 ppm with the average of 63.15 ppm noted in the Kayamkulam estuary (Table. 5.4). The concentration of Co observed in the study area was higher than the upper continental crust (UCC) value. In the surface sediments the significant enrichment of Co was from natural sources and was supplemented by an adequate supply of fluvial sediments from the mainland (Fig. 5.8). Similar observations were noted out in estuarine systems in the state of Andhra Pradesh, India (Reddy *et al.*, 2016).

Stations including Kayamkulam, Anchuthengu and Kappil – Hariharapuram estuaries fall in same group with pertinent point sources such as thermal power plant, fish processing plants and harbour. Robin *et al.*, 2012 states that in the low salinity ranges elevated concentrations of trace elements in the estuarine environments were accredited to remineralization from sediment substrate and organic matter. In the process of trace element accumulation and exchange between sediments and water column in the river – sea water intermixing zone, chief controlling factor is particle size (Biksham *et al.*, 1991).

**Table. 5.1** Fe, Mn and trace element concentration (all values in ppm) in the surface sediments, Kadinamkulam estuary, Kerala, India

| Sample No | Cr | Cu | Pb | Co | Ni | Zn | Mn | Fe |
|---|---|---|---|---|---|---|---|---|
| 1 | 251.66 | 163.95 | 47.90 | 33.68 | 151.30 | 155.76 | 108.64 | 10887.63 |
| 2 | 165.03 | 108.58 | 62.07 | 33.66 | 104.78 | 173.84 | 91.95 | 7681.37 |
| 3 | 11.91 | 5.97 | 42.05 | 1.04 | 19.87 | 13.70 | 887.59 | 17795.70 |
| 4 | 208.60 | 38.89 | 75.20 | 37.02 | 111.44 | 224.03 | 213.64 | 16064.54 |
| 5 | 179.50 | 55.26 | 69.83 | 36.42 | 101.32 | 178.61 | 136.35 | 11686.04 |
| 6 | 259.25 | 74.63 | 88.02 | 38.31 | 117.95 | 170.49 | 528.70 | 23377.84 |
| 7 | 237.99 | 134.36 | 79.76 | 36.18 | 109.87 | 190.27 | 216.03 | 19440.65 |
| 8 | 283.83 | 54.39 | 79.72 | 37.48 | 119.57 | 138.99 | 224.99 | 25492.58 |
| 9 | 283.93 | 34.16 | 76.11 | 30.07 | 108.40 | 86.34 | 268.16 | 24624.95 |
| 10 | 262.95 | 56.09 | 83.17 | 28.94 | 107.99 | 116.03 | 328.38 | 22983.94 |
| 11 | 396.18 | 37.86 | 91.93 | 38.31 | 141.01 | 106.83 | 287.30 | 26332.91 |
| 12 | 279.07 | 48.94 | 80.81 | 37.19 | 94.86 | 92.21 | 197.13 | 27762.27 |
| 13 | 235.01 | 51.97 | 83.47 | 34.08 | 102.79 | 90.45 | 238.72 | 24037.15 |
| 14 | 271.53 | 25.90 | 74.96 | 30.29 | 131.67 | 75.31 | 149.32 | 13704.52 |
| 15 | 268.71 | 62.16 | 73.35 | 30.93 | 111.78 | 182.43 | 107.84 | 22899.21 |
| 16 | 307.23 | 31.15 | 73.50 | 30.74 | 137.30 | 97.46 | 249.80 | 23188.66 |
| 17 | 299.38 | 82.43 | 84.37 | 38.71 | 122.34 | 176.95 | 263.83 | 31438.17 |
| 18 | 284.66 | 100.95 | 77.80 | 34.09 | 112.76 | 109.93 | 203.84 | 20293.74 |
| 19 | 180.22 | 28.23 | 74.19 | 31.14 | 78.78 | 77.38 | 138.29 | 13199.32 |
| 20 | 226.90 | 126.31 | 72.30 | 31.23 | 108.38 | 179.36 | 185.85 | 17174.25 |
| 21 | 256.11 | 74.77 | 89.76 | 29.50 | 106.64 | 139.23 | 165.80 | 15670.50 |
| 22 | 274.74 | 63.73 | 94.23 | 41.26 | 118.30 | 119.71 | 219.81 | 22288.36 |
| 23 | 362.57 | 70.44 | 84.60 | 39.29 | 163.75 | 116.66 | 175.01 | 19532.15 |
| **Avg** | **251.61** | **66.57** | **76.48** | **33.02** | **112.30** | **130.96** | **242.91** | **19893.76** |
| **Max** | **396.18** | **163.95** | **94.23** | **41.26** | **163.75** | **224.03** | **887.59** | **31438.17** |
| **Min** | **11.91** | **5.97** | **42.05** | **1.04** | **19.87** | **13.70** | **91.95** | **7681.37** |

**Table. 5.2** Fe, Mn and trace element concentration (all values in ppm) in the surface sediments, Anchuthengu estuary, Kerala, India

| Sample No | Cr | Cu | Pb | Co | Ni | Zn | Mn | Fe |
|---|---|---|---|---|---|---|---|---|
| 24 | 283.27 | 37.30 | 53.38 | 36.31 | 99.11 | 96.26 | 311.12 | 28761.84 |
| 25 | 326.16 | 108.61 | 61.11 | 36.90 | 105.68 | 185.53 | 265.74 | 45798.75 |
| 26 | 308.93 | 182.97 | 71.37 | 37.48 | 99.04 | 165.06 | 234.38 | 42362.91 |
| 27 | 282.93 | 33.67 | 63.65 | 35.91 | 122.21 | 112.16 | 242.63 | 35039.31 |
| 28 | 211.68 | 21.45 | 47.60 | 27.73 | 72.80 | 62.20 | 256.27 | 15754.99 |
| 29 | 271.52 | 48.38 | 48.80 | 33.22 | 85.30 | 98.68 | 125.09 | 27421.21 |
| 30 | 223.53 | 17.47 | 44.73 | 35.32 | 96.71 | 73.18 | 147.01 | 16545.42 |
| 31 | 540.21 | 92.50 | 38.70 | 45.40 | 338.68 | 97.35 | 187.55 | 14124.28 |
| 32 | 193.42 | 16.91 | 41.96 | 35.07 | 117.30 | 64.54 | 134.64 | 12914.99 |
| 33 | 175.51 | 139.37 | 47.34 | 35.46 | 75.52 | 133.32 | 228.75 | 14932.08 |
| 34 | 229.25 | 60.90 | 50.95 | 37.91 | 109.68 | 137.83 | 113.46 | 12950.32 |
| 35 | 197.10 | 126.82 | 70.54 | 35.98 | 77.32 | 121.69 | 253.02 | 17924.95 |
| 36 | 308.95 | 37.52 | 57.17 | 37.04 | 125.95 | 101.91 | 110.66 | 22550.78 |
| 37 | 263.61 | 35.46 | 77.07 | 38.67 | 119.78 | 83.03 | 68.19 | 27216.58 |
| 38 | 249.31 | 19.59 | 65.42 | 39.02 | 110.30 | 70.17 | 110.65 | 16030.92 |
| 39 | 204.21 | 114.67 | 62.06 | 39.36 | 97.19 | 159.69 | 196.90 | 15832.99 |
| 40 | 269.04 | 119.76 | 67.95 | 39.84 | 99.33 | 135.09 | 316.93 | 29595.47 |
| 41 | 333.99 | 40.02 | 71.62 | 35.05 | 139.89 | 145.89 | 133.07 | 23009.03 |
| 42 | 292.52 | 39.88 | 71.54 | 42.14 | 120.26 | 115.98 | 229.27 | 28612.67 |
| 43 | 219.99 | 167.39 | 65.64 | 39.46 | 104.45 | 187.54 | 203.24 | 16418.38 |
| 44 | 250.34 | 23.40 | 62.42 | 40.33 | 123.24 | 82.55 | 178.26 | 158639.33 |
| 45 | 239.31 | 23.21 | 62.51 | 33.36 | 119.05 | 83.25 | 94.28 | 69003.19 |
| 46 | 172.46 | 71.23 | 69.16 | 30.49 | 97.93 | 74.52 | 215.87 | 15854.06 |
| 47 | 298.13 | 70.71 | 103.65 | 45.50 | 143.97 | 139.02 | 312.64 | 28320.79 |
| 48 | 274.33 | 38.53 | 112.01 | 44.38 | 134.79 | 111.06 | 1063.84 | 21895.48 |
| 49 | 310.84 | 173.30 | 105.53 | 42.97 | 127.04 | 237.03 | 541.68 | 36907.27 |
| 50 | 361.93 | 120.49 | 110.98 | 47.08 | 145.61 | 225.62 | 451.17 | 33444.98 |
| 51 | 269.21 | 42.36 | 114.81 | 46.18 | 112.15 | 122.28 | 387.43 | 29078.03 |
| 52 | 266.86 | 105.08 | 99.76 | 41.03 | 118.16 | 123.05 | 456.32 | 35293.70 |
| 53 | 298.70 | 68.13 | 108.35 | 44.31 | 127.85 | 137.79 | 425.72 | 36591.66 |
| 54 | 283.12 | 38.95 | 109.28 | 42.23 | 125.61 | 116.60 | 547.30 | 21405.36 |
| 55 | 312.22 | 43.35 | 116.55 | 48.22 | 139.57 | 122.72 | 404.36 | 36727.96 |
| **Avg** | **272.58** | **71.23** | **73.55** | **39.04** | **119.73** | **122.58** | **279.61** | **30842.49** |
| **Max** | **540.21** | **182.97** | **116.55** | **48.22** | **338.68** | **237.03** | **1063.84** | **158639.33** |
| **Min** | **172.46** | **16.91** | **38.70** | **27.73** | **72.80** | **62.20** | **68.19** | **12914.99** |

Department of Geology, UNOM

**Table. 5.3** Fe, Mn and trace element concentration (all values in ppm) in the surface sediments, Kappil - Hariharapuram estuary, Kerala, India

| Sample No | Cr | Cu | Pb | Co | Ni | Zn | Mn | Fe |
|---|---|---|---|---|---|---|---|---|
| 56 | 311.60 | 69.68 | 94.62 | 34.61 | 141.58 | 96.18 | 417.56 | 22740.73 |
| 57 | 287.66 | 85.14 | 99.73 | 41.63 | 136.72 | 117.44 | 323.70 | 28772.47 |
| 58 | 310.97 | 41.09 | 99.43 | 44.85 | 137.67 | 89.36 | 454.86 | 39169.99 |
| 59 | 315.09 | 38.17 | 108.10 | 35.41 | 128.44 | 157.13 | 286.27 | 35962.34 |
| 60 | 340.41 | 165.52 | 97.47 | 37.88 | 161.13 | 135.69 | 191.64 | 22586.82 |
| 61 | 327.67 | 82.95 | 101.28 | 35.33 | 161.18 | 157.67 | 228.26 | 26305.26 |
| 62 | 285.13 | 132.83 | 103.67 | 33.18 | 125.68 | 209.42 | 768.58 | 26020.79 |
| 63 | 378.29 | 168.30 | 105.36 | 44.32 | 139.90 | 268.86 | 378.52 | 47533.91 |
| 64 | 281.80 | 35.30 | 95.14 | 36.85 | 124.03 | 101.41 | 405.34 | 20627.45 |
| 65 | 303.15 | 87.97 | 99.25 | 38.45 | 131.34 | 158.33 | 415.41 | 31402.43 |
| 66 | 302.02 | 98.32 | 90.81 | 34.09 | 137.63 | 129.92 | 153.40 | 30618.53 |
| 67 | 204.97 | 335.04 | 88.54 | 28.24 | 103.83 | 369.61 | 237.69 | 18570.28 |
| 68 | 230.20 | 129.82 | 88.02 | 33.67 | 107.36 | 272.93 | 270.72 | 14204.11 |
| 69 | 237.05 | 607.29 | 99.34 | 37.57 | 110.64 | 352.91 | 274.30 | 22368.75 |
| 70 | 315.25 | 107.60 | 101.98 | 42.41 | 141.86 | 209.52 | 267.40 | 30042.35 |
| 71 | 282.02 | 298.60 | 97.66 | 40.17 | 123.31 | 341.72 | 307.91 | 33776.37 |
| 72 | 237.14 | 89.38 | 76.32 | 29.88 | 99.58 | 149.38 | 221.65 | 15557.50 |
| 73 | 341.58 | 93.17 | 90.43 | 37.87 | 180.67 | 142.82 | 231.27 | 27120.29 |
| 74 | 263.77 | 193.07 | 94.06 | 37.51 | 113.85 | 324.46 | 180.20 | 21056.54 |
| 75 | 303.86 | 145.69 | 107.91 | 42.09 | 116.48 | 307.28 | 253.10 | 39077.79 |
| 76 | 247.15 | 92.51 | 73.34 | 29.02 | 113.02 | 116.58 | 191.60 | 19503.33 |
| 77 | 319.67 | 143.10 | 105.33 | 38.08 | 129.72 | 127.01 | 287.65 | 27010.68 |
| 78 | 210.94 | 76.53 | 98.77 | 12.50 | 92.33 | 83.46 | 255.14 | 14660.31 |
| 79 | 230.42 | 136.63 | 84.74 | 32.84 | 119.00 | 236.32 | 168.90 | 17626.17 |
| 80 | 203.30 | 40.39 | 89.70 | 28.55 | 106.94 | 65.50 | 146.37 | 16796.65 |
| 81 | 296.81 | 119.40 | 95.91 | 26.16 | 120.56 | 165.31 | 273.68 | 29166.81 |
| 82 | 295.83 | 267.59 | 102.69 | 36.47 | 134.30 | 299.61 | 311.64 | 24726.47 |
| Avg | 283.84 | 143.74 | 95.91 | 35.17 | 127.36 | 192.07 | 292.69 | 26037.23 |
| Max | 378.29 | 607.29 | 108.10 | 44.85 | 180.67 | 369.61 | 768.58 | 47533.91 |
| Min | 203.30 | 35.30 | 73.34 | 12.50 | 92.33 | 65.50 | 146.37 | 14204.11 |

**Table. 5.4** Fe, Mn and trace element concentration (all values in ppm) in the surface sediments, Kayamkulam estuary, Kerala, India

| Sample No | Cr | Cu | Pb | Co | Ni | Zn | Mn | Fe |
|---|---|---|---|---|---|---|---|---|
| 83 | 206.19 | 39.86 | 87.16 | 30.94 | 98.40 | 198.78 | 280.85 | 16392.08 |
| 84 | 559.08 | 38.80 | 91.58 | 60.23 | 262.06 | 179.76 | 443.27 | 35992.59 |
| 85 | 277.73 | 28.63 | 107.68 | 49.07 | 119.62 | 160.59 | 322.66 | 23151.31 |
| 86 | 350.04 | 28.81 | 92.55 | 72.84 | 150.66 | 143.90 | 348.69 | 25858.25 |
| 87 | 238.15 | 34.68 | 85.30 | 31.92 | 111.42 | 141.24 | 309.67 | 19578.78 |
| 88 | 504.58 | 35.74 | 88.78 | 20.38 | 91.31 | 105.75 | 370.34 | 22988.09 |
| 89 | 366.73 | 14.85 | 86.81 | 98.70 | 144.72 | 57.86 | 248.32 | 12129.48 |
| 90 | 232.61 | 11.86 | 84.74 | 152.13 | 91.04 | 78.05 | 269.23 | 21165.20 |
| 91 | 260.27 | 11.84 | 82.41 | 75.24 | 139.04 | 76.96 | 202.21 | 10293.55 |
| 92 | 243.49 | 11.14 | 90.08 | 70.51 | 88.75 | 55.93 | 178.94 | 8086.75 |
| 93 | 255.54 | 16.78 | 94.37 | 79.98 | 107.88 | 84.57 | 266.75 | 18852.45 |
| 94 | 352.20 | 52.62 | 98.94 | 38.44 | 131.06 | 148.47 | 322.72 | 22474.94 |
| 95 | 307.74 | 22.89 | 99.04 | 34.12 | 104.30 | 104.92 | 338.42 | 29457.38 |
| 96 | 764.33 | 49.38 | 95.40 | 65.51 | 450.98 | 116.08 | 307.77 | 27302.99 |
| 97 | 354.03 | 32.31 | 102.16 | 44.94 | 129.13 | 120.82 | 375.35 | 36305.73 |
| 98 | 350.50 | 37.92 | 94.77 | 34.63 | 123.90 | 117.52 | 374.21 | 40518.15 |
| 99 | 259.04 | 29.75 | 88.60 | 19.28 | 89.35 | 65.11 | 336.31 | 18194.73 |
| 100 | 335.09 | 28.39 | 96.06 | 48.39 | 114.11 | 111.64 | 353.29 | 36299.11 |
| 101 | 385.28 | 30.71 | 100.22 | 49.92 | 132.34 | 133.53 | 345.06 | 42163.35 |
| 102 | 220.71 | 9.91 | 90.90 | 80.47 | 93.43 | 74.96 | 257.01 | 15418.52 |
| 103 | 262.86 | 11.74 | 94.24 | 109.85 | 98.01 | 80.71 | 363.11 | 20799.66 |
| 104 | 372.08 | 22.90 | 86.82 | 61.84 | 119.54 | 104.04 | 324.57 | 32602.41 |
| 105 | 300.28 | 16.95 | 82.40 | 67.10 | 102.30 | 86.63 | 310.43 | 24433.00 |
| 106 | 308.23 | 13.28 | 89.79 | 118.47 | 139.41 | 98.76 | 333.34 | 21313.55 |
| 107 | 321.37 | 11.58 | 94.65 | 100.47 | 130.10 | 76.87 | 202.31 | 12168.07 |
| 108 | 382.93 | 27.60 | 95.42 | 63.82 | 202.20 | 128.58 | 407.67 | 32087.60 |
| 109 | 268.27 | 25.57 | 93.33 | 33.91 | 128.45 | 99.15 | 283.79 | 19226.95 |
| 110 | 230.64 | 12.76 | 82.79 | 74.71 | 106.44 | 80.76 | 268.94 | 15363.43 |
| 111 | 351.30 | 18.25 | 100.68 | 43.45 | 118.30 | 92.78 | 442.33 | 22795.32 |
| Avg | 331.77 | 25.09 | 92.33 | 63.15 | 135.11 | 107.75 | 316.81 | 23565.98 |
| Max | 764.33 | 52.62 | 107.68 | 152.13 | 450.98 | 198.78 | 443.27 | 42163.35 |
| Min | 206.19 | 9.91 | 82.40 | 19.28 | 88.75 | 55.93 | 178.94 | 8086.75 |

Department of Geology, UNOM

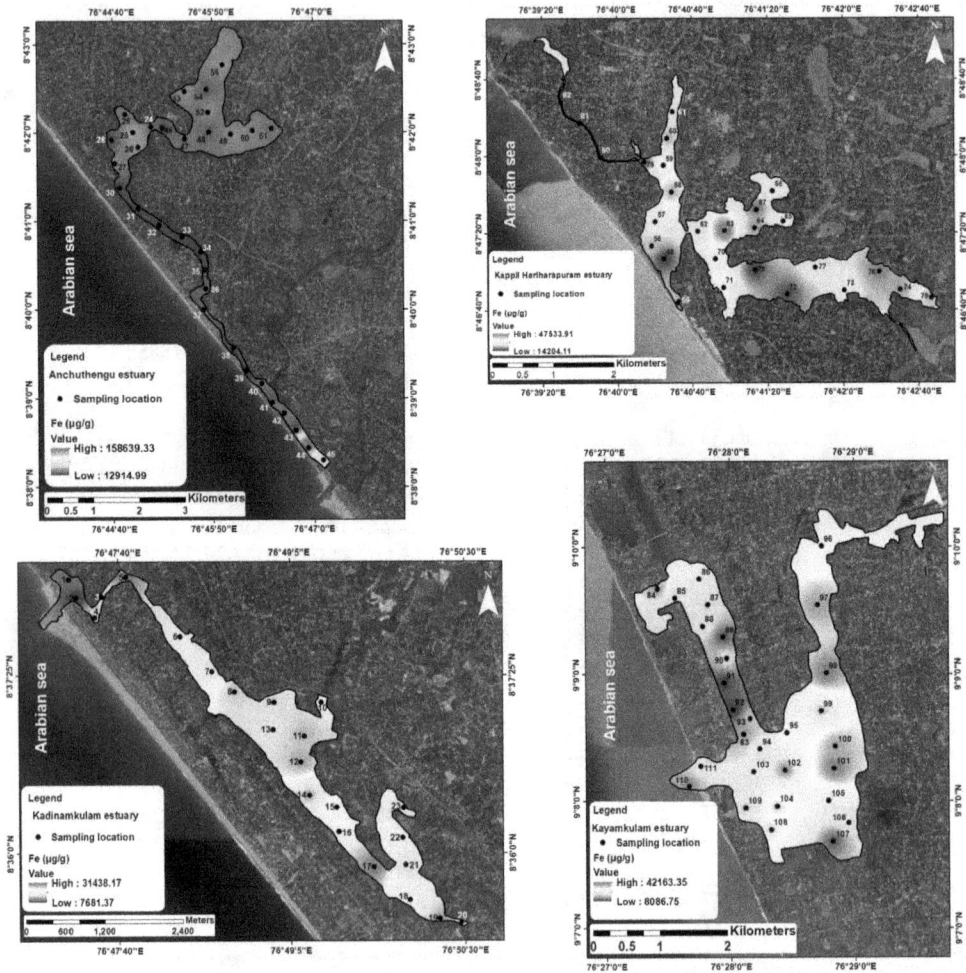

**Fig. 5.1** Spatial distribution map of the element Fe (in µg/g), in the surface sediments, selected estuaries in Kerala, India

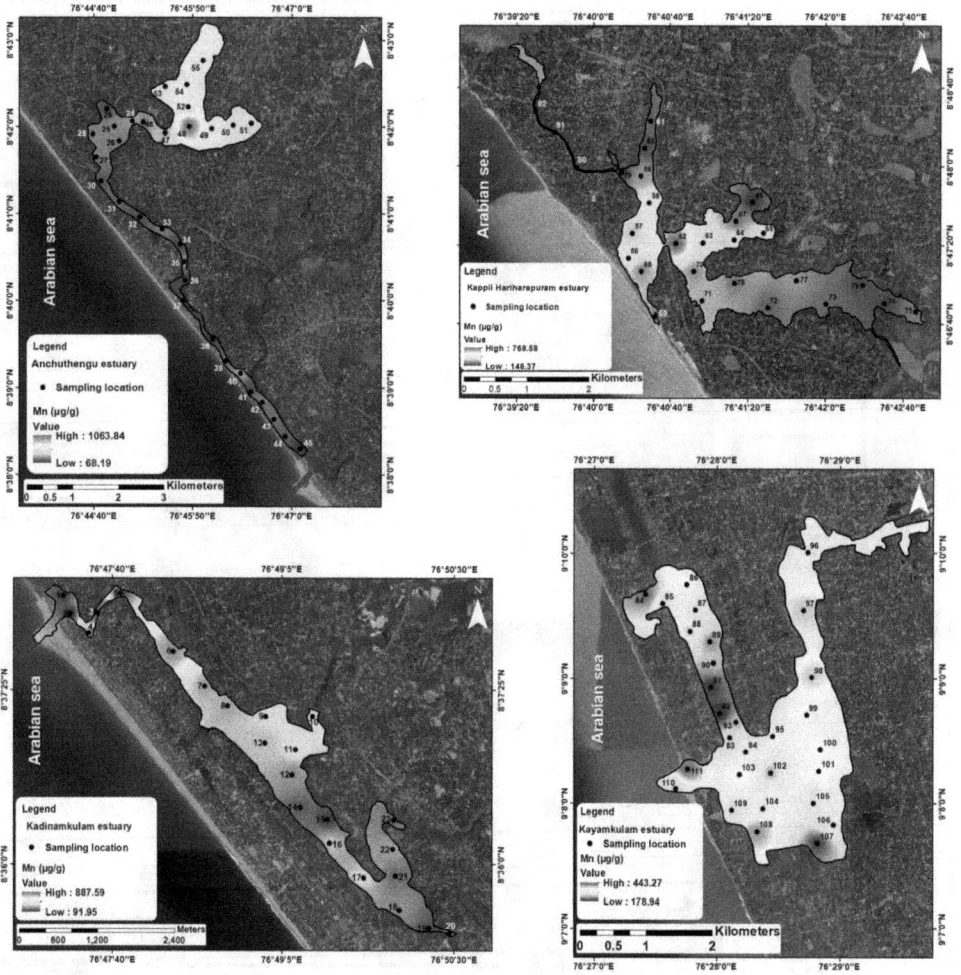

**Fig. 5.2** Spatial distribution map of the element Mn (in µg/g), in the surface sediments, selected estuaries in Kerala, India

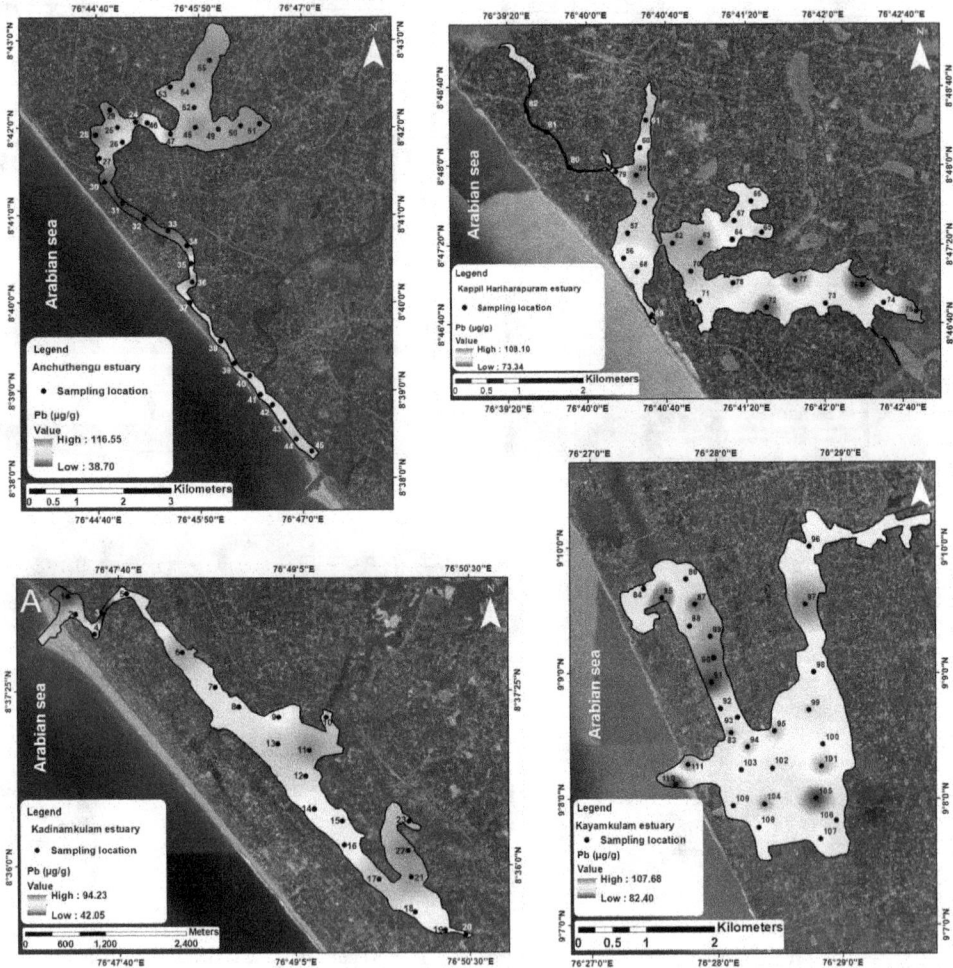

**Fig. 5.3** Spatial distribution map of the element Pb (in µg/g), in the surface sediments, selected estuaries in Kerala, India

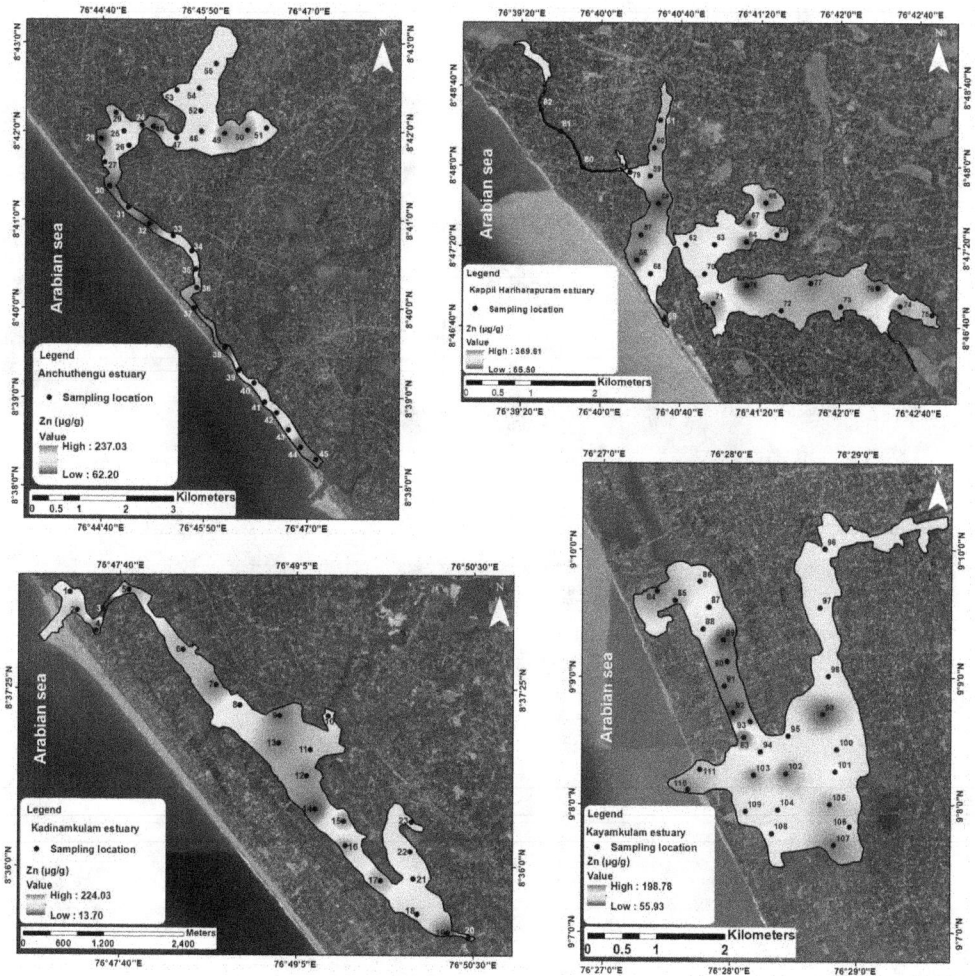

**Fig. 5.4** Spatial distribution map of the element Zn (in µg/g), in the surface sediments,
selected estuaries in Kerala, India

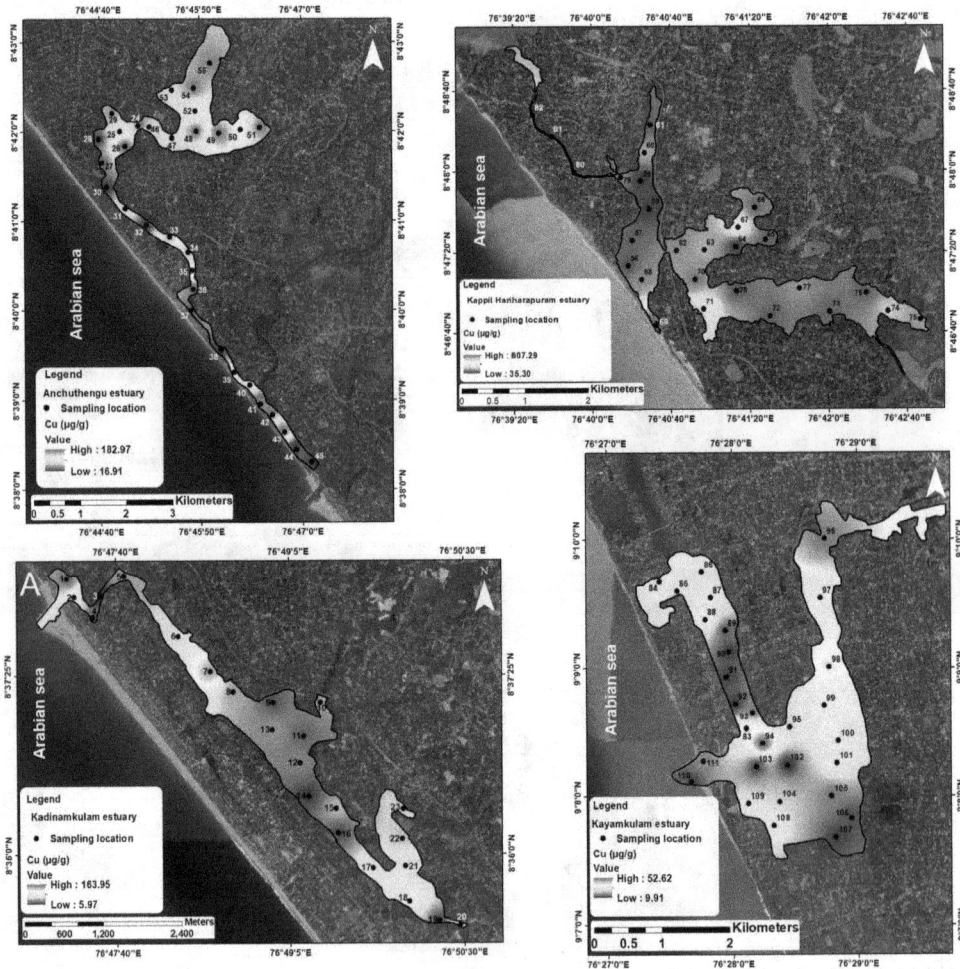

**Fig. 5.5** Spatial distribution map of the element Cu (in μg/g), in the surface sediments, selected estuaries in Kerala, India

Department of Geology, UNOM

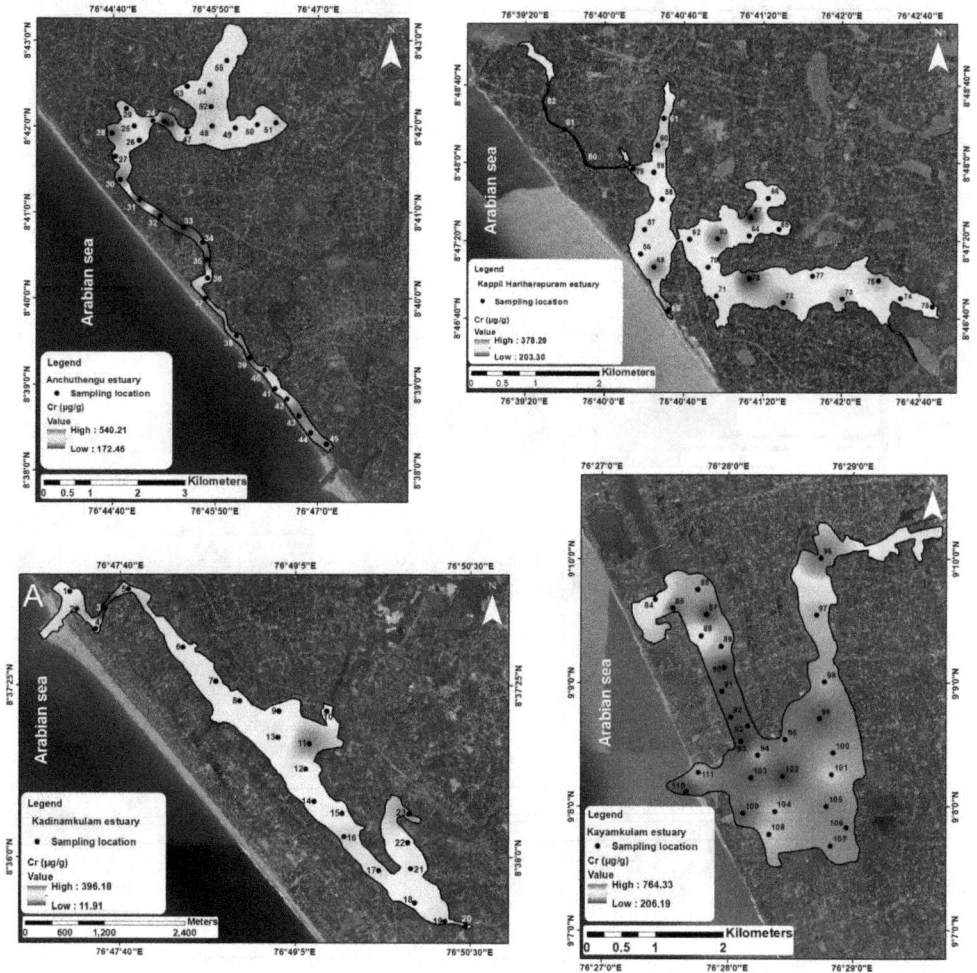

**Fig. 5.6** Spatial distribution map of the element Cr (in μg/g), in the surface sediments, selected estuaries in Kerala, India

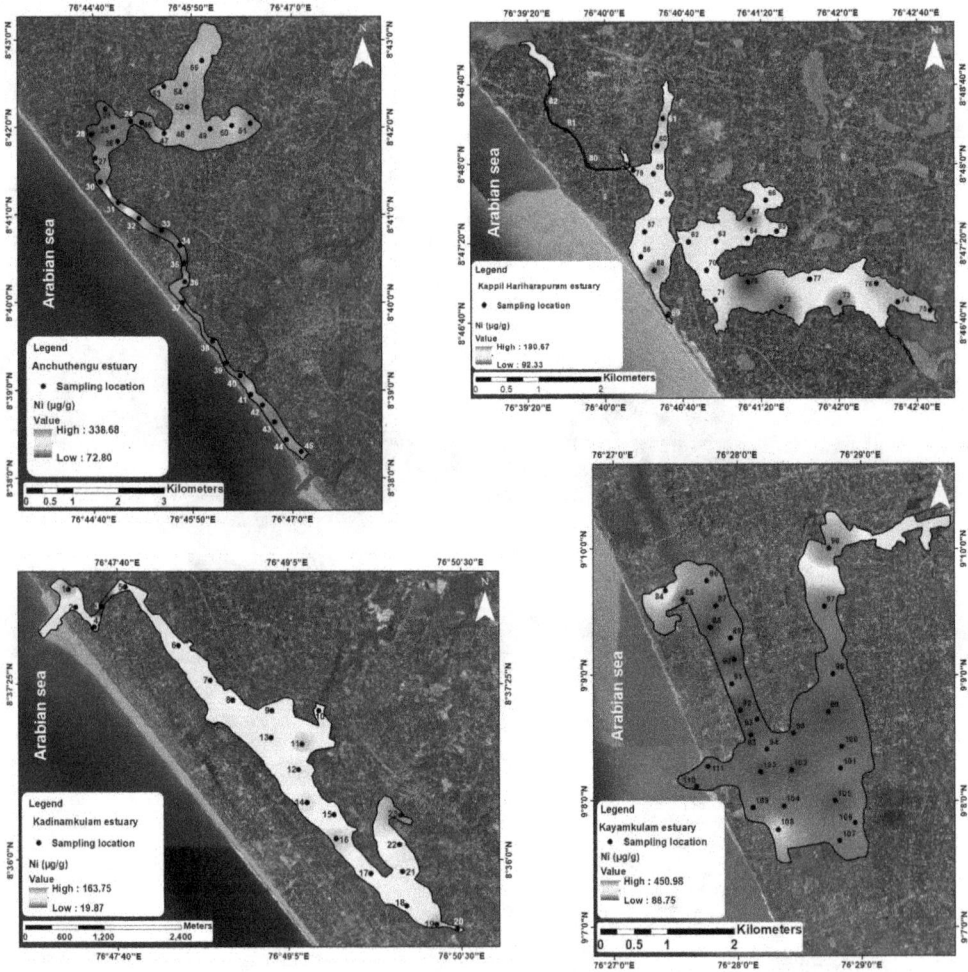

**Fig. 5.7** Spatial distribution map of the element Ni (in µg/g), in the surface sediments, selected estuaries in Kerala, India

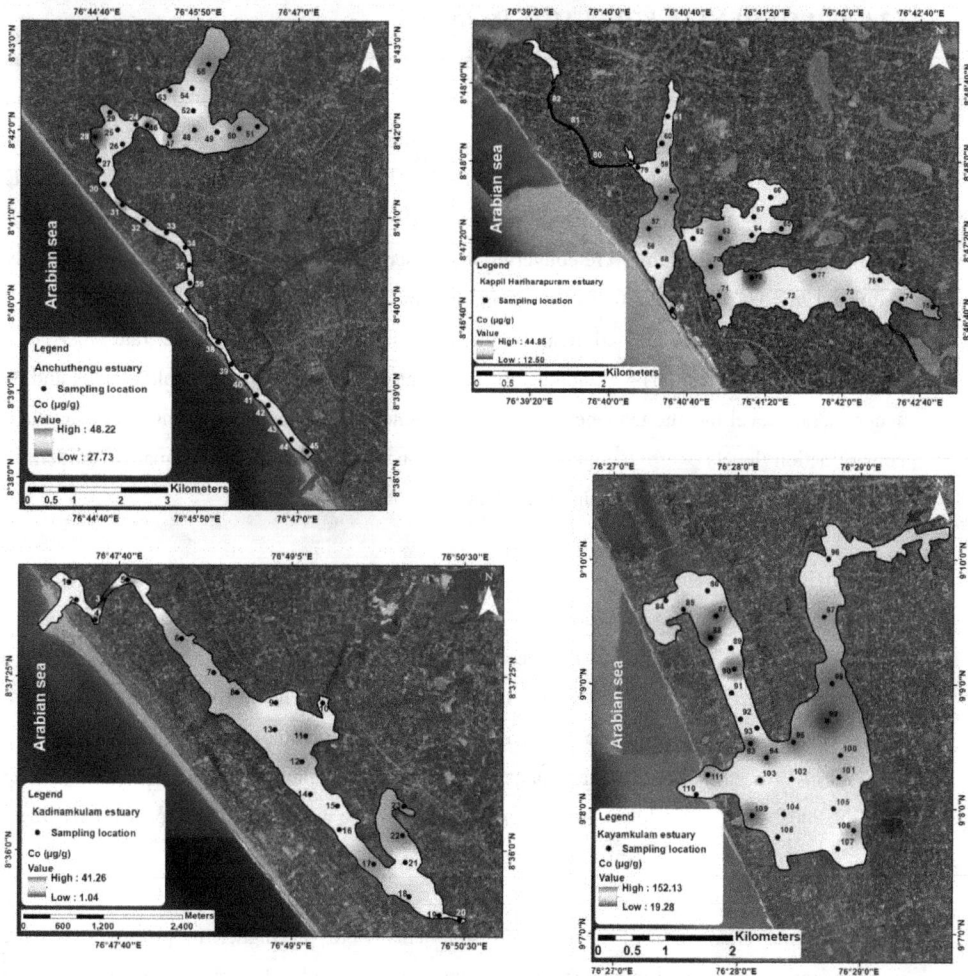

**Fig. 5.8** Spatial distribution map of the element Co (in µg/g), in the surface sediments, selected estuaries in Kerala, India

## 5.3 ENVIRONMENTAL POLLUTION IMPACTS

Assessment of lagoonal and coastal environment based on the trace elements includes various calculation methods (Muller, 1969; Hakanson, 1980). The present study is systemized to compare the trace metal enrichment in the surficial sediments from the selected estuaries in Kerala using various pollution indices. In order to quantify the metal enrichment degree in sediments several estimating methods for pollution impact have been proposed (Ridgway and Schimmield, 2002). The calculated results were converted into descriptive ranges/bands of pollution intensity (Muller, 1969; Hakanson, 1980; Salomons and Forstner, 1984). Langston *et al.* (2010) discussed that the adverse effects of sediment pollution is seen from the tolerance rate, resistance mechanisms in organism. The guidelines for sediment quality based on the contaminants and its accumulation level has the tendency to impact the potentials of sediment. Hence the calculated contamination levels were compared with reference data and sediment quality guidelines (Vetrimurugan *et al.*, 2019; Hussain *et al.*, 2020).

### 5.3.1 Enrichment Factor (EF)

EF was determined to discover if the metal levels in the sediments of selected estuarine sediments and its surrounding marine environment were of anthropogenic origin (e.g., contamination). In order to study the metal enrichment and heavy metal contamination, the metal Al was used as normalized metal (Selvaraj *et al.*, 2004). Various authors have successfully utilized Fe to normalize heavy metals contaminants, since iron is abundant metal in the earth crust (Zhang and Liu, 2002; Feng *et al.*, 2004). In the present study also, Fe was adopted as a conservative tracer to distinguish natural from anthropogenic components.

Natural abundance of elements in sediments were far higher in proportion to the anthropogenic inputs, for compensating grain size variations and sediment composition variation the metal Fe is applied (Loring and Rantala, 1992). In this computation, the ratio between metal/Fe$_{sample}$ and metal/Fe $_{local\ background}$ was applied as a normalization value to evaluate the sediment quality (Saravanan *et al.*, 2018, Hussain *et al.*, 2020). The classification of enrichment classes was classified as (Acevedo-Figueroa *et al.*, 2006):

> If, EF < 1 indicates no enrichment (natural enrichment),
> If, EF 1-3 for minor enrichment,
> If, EF 3-5 for moderate enrichment;
> If, EF 5-10 for moderately severe enrichment,
> If, EF 10-25 for severe enrichment,
> If, EF 25-50 for very severe enrichment, and
> If, EF >50 for extremely severe enrichment.

All of the metal enrichment in this investigation was concluded to be natural enrichment to extremely severe enrichment. The above-mentioned metal enrichment trend shows natural to extremely severe enrichment in the estuarine sediments derived from the geogenic process to severe anthropogenic influences, whereas Pb and Cr showing moderately severe to severe enrichment. These two metals infer their origin is from anthropogenic sources such as atmospheric deposition, fishing activities and anti-fouling agents used as coatings in boats. The enrichment values changing from each metal and location. The values of EF in the selected estuaries in the following decreasing order Cr > Pb > Mn > Cu > Zn > Ni > Co for Kadinamkulam estuary (Table. 5.5; Fig. 5.9 & 5.10), Cr >Pb >Mn > Cu > Ni >Zn > Co for Anchuthengu estuary (Table. 5.7; Fig. 5.11 & 5.12), Cr > Pb > Cu > Mn > Zn > Ni > Co for Kappil - Hariharapuram estuary (Table. 5.9; Fig. 5.13 & 5.14) and Cr > Pb > Mn > Ni > Zn > Co > Cu for Kayamkulam estuary (Table. 5.11; Fig. 5.15 & 5.16), respectively. The most dominant trace elements enriched in the selected four estuaries are Cr and Pb. Most probably these elements are derived from several activities of thermal power plant, fisheries and atmospheric deposition along the estuaries and coast.

## 5.3.2 Contamination Factor (CF)

Sediments have been generally used as environmental indicators due to its ability to trace the source of contamination and in monitoring the contaminants it is well documented. Trace elements play a key role in assessing the pollutants in sediments those are readily prone to aquatic organisms, physico-chemical variations initiated by the releasing of metals again into the aqueous medium (Jayaprakash *et al.*, 2008). Trace metals have adverse and harmful effect on the environment, contamination factor is used in order to express the level of contamination in the sediments (Pekey *et al.*, 2004). The ratio between metal content of the sample to respective metals background value for individual metals and sampling stations was employed to calculate the CF of the sediments. The classification of contamination factor classes is classified as (Tomlinson *et al.,* 1980):

> ➤ From $1 \leq CF$ low contamination factor
> ➤ If $1 \leq CF < 3$ moderate contamination factor
> ➤ If $3 \leq CF < 6$ considerable contamination factor
> ➤ If $\geq 6$ very high contamination factor

Background value for this calculation was taken from lowest value of trace element concentration from the sediment core sample from the Anchuthengu estuary (Jeshma, 2020). The contamination factor of the investigated selected estuarine surface sediments shows following decreasing order of its distribution: Kadinamkulam estuary Cr > Pb > Mn > Zn > Cu > Ni > Fe > Co (Table. 5.5; Fig. 5.17 & 5.18); Anchuthengu estuary Cr > Pb > Mn > Cu > Zn > Ni > Fe > Co (Table.5.7; Fig. 5.19 & 5.20); Kappil - Hariharapuram Cr > Pb > Cu > Mn > Zn > Ni > Fe > Co (Table. 5.9; Fig. 5.21 & 5.22) and Kayamkulam estuary Cr > Pb > Mn > Ni > Zn > Co > Fe > Cu (Table. 5.11; Fig. 5.23 to 5.24). The most dominant trace elements contaminating sediments in the four estuaries are Cr and Pb.

### 5.3.3 Geo-accumulation Index ($I_{geo}$)

It is difficult to assess the metal contamination in the marine and marginal marine sediments. However, various researchers reported the consequences of differences in analytical procedures between background data and studied samples in the marine and coastal environments. In order to evaluate the metal pollution extent, Geo-accumulation index ($I_{geo}$) was applied as normalizing factor for trace metal concentration (Muller, 1979). Determination of the degree of contamination by this calculation was made on the comparison of present element concentration with the global standard levels or pre-industrial values (Rubio *et al.,* 2000). The $I_{geo}$ level in the surface sediments of four selected estuaries on Kerala's south west coast was enumerated using local background data as a normalising data in this study (Hussain *et al.,* 2020). To evaluate the sediment quality, Muller specified the following ranges. Igeo value and Sediment Quality ranges were as follows

> If, $I_{geo}$ < 0, Unpolluted;

> If, $I_{geo}$ 0-1, From unpolluted to moderately polluted;

> If, $I_{geo}$ 1-2, Moderately polluted;

> If, $I_{geo}$ 2-3, From moderately polluted to strongly polluted;

> If, $I_{geo}$ 3-4, Strongly polluted;

> If, $I_{geo}$ 4-5, From strongly to extremely polluted;

> If, $I_{geo}$ >5, Extremely polluted.

The results of the study suggests that the $I_{geo}$ values found to be variating from unpolluted to extremely polluted and that too changing from location to location and also metal to metal, in all four estuaries. The mean of the $I_{geo}$ values of the sediments was moderately to strongly polluted by Cr and Pb in Kadinamkulam estuary (Table. 5.6; Fig. 5.25 to 5.26) and Anchuthengu estuary (Table. 5.8; Fig. 5.27 to 5.28); by Cr, Pb, Cu and Mn in Kappil- Hariharapuram estuary (Table. 5.10; Fig. 5.29 to 5.30). and by Cr, Pb and Mn in Kayamkulam estuary (Table. 5.12; Fig. 5.31 to 5.32). Whereas the sediments were unpolluted to moderately polluted by other metals like Fe, Co, Ni and Zn in all the four estuaries.

### 5.3.4 Pollution Load Index (PLI)

To evaluate the degree of metal contamination in estuary sediments, Tomlinson et al., 1980 used a simplistic method based on the Pollution Load Index (PLI).

The equation was used to compute the sediment PLI.

$$CF = C_{metal} / C_{background}$$
$$PLI = n (CF1 \times CF2 \times CF3 \times \ldots\ldots \quad CFn)$$

**Where,**

CF - contamination factor

$C_{metal}$ - concentration of pollutant in sediment

$C_{background}$ - background value for the metal

n - number of metals

**PLI status:** PLI > 1 polluted; < 1 no pollution

The PLI of the studied estuaries ranging 1.23 to 5.42 in Kadinamkulam estuary indicating sediments were polluted by the metal concentration (Table. 5.6; Fig. 5.33), PLI ranging from 2.48 to 7.30 in Anchuthengu estuary indicating the sediments were polluted by the metal concentration (Table. 5.8; Fig. 5.33), PLI values of all the sediments in Kappil- Hariharapuram estuary exceeding 1 indicating pollution by the metal concentration (Table. 5.10; Fig. 5.33) and PLI values of all the sediments in Kayamkulam estuary exceeding 1 indicating pollution by the metal concentration (Table. 5.12; Fig. 5.33). Anthropogenic influences majorly control the levels of PLI of the sediments. The investigation show pollution in all the samples with that we conclude the present environment is considered to be polluted based on the PLI study.

### 5.3.5 Sediment Pollution Index (SPI)

Singh et al. (2002) suggested the sediment pollution index SPI as a way to assess sediment quality in terms of trace metal concentration and metal toxicity. The SPI can be denoted as:

$$SPI=\sum \frac{EFm \times Wm}{\sum Wm}$$

$$EF_m = \frac{Cn}{CR}$$

Here, Wm is the toxicity weight, and EFm is the ratio between the measured metal concentration (Cn) and the background metal concentration (CR). According to Hakanson (1980), Cr and Zn have a toxicity weight of 1, Cu and Ni have a toxicity weight of 2, Pb has a toxicity weight of 5, and Cd has a toxicity weight of 30. Based on this pollution classification, the SPI was classified as following:

➢ From 0 to 2 = natural sediment,
➢ From 2 to 5 = low polluted sediment,
➢ From 5 to 10 = moderately polluted sediment,
➢ From 10 to 20 = highly polluted sediment, and
➢ Greater than 20 = dangerous sediment.

The investigation based on the SPI shows that sediments in Kadinamkulam estuary ranges from natural sediments to moderately polluted sediments (Table. 5.6; Fig. 5.34), in Anchuthengu estuary SPI values ranges from low polluted to moderately polluted sediments (Table. 5.8; Fig. 5.34), in Kappil- Hariharapuram estuary SPI value ranges from moderately polluted to highly polluted sediments (Table. 5.10; Fig. 5.34) and in Kayamkulam estuary the SPI value ranges from moderately polluted to highly polluted sediments (Table. 5.12; Fig 5.34).

### 5.3.6 Potential Ecological Risk Index (PERI)

Toxic metals resulting from anthropogenic activity are the most common environmental pollutants. Intake of these trace metals, which are normally hazardous compounds to living creatures, worsens the undesirable health consequences caused by their existence in the environment (Rahman *et al.,* 2014). Hakanson (1980) proposed a potential ecological risk index. PERI uses ecological analysis to assess the impact of heavy metals on the ecosystem (Guo et al., 2010; Saeedi et al., 2012). The following formulae can be used to compute the risk index (RI).

$$C_f^i = C_D^i / C_B^i$$

$$E_r^i = T_r^i \times C_f^i$$

$$RI = \sum_{i=1}^{m} E_r^i$$

Here, RI is the sum of individual heavy metal potential risks, $E_r^i$ is the individual heavy metal potential risk, $T_r^i$ is the toxic-response factor for a selected metal (Hakanson, 1980), Cf I is the contamination factor, $C_D^i$ is the current concentration of metals in sediments, and $C_B^i$ is the background concentration record of metal in crust (Taylor, 1964 The toxic response factors for the studied trace elements are denoted as 5 for Cu, Pb, Co and Ni; 2 for Cr, 1 for Zn and Mn. Background value for this calculation was taken from lowest value of trace element concentration from the sediment core sample from the Anchuthengu estuary (Jeshma 2020). Hakanson (1980) classified five group of ecological risk (Ei) grades and four group of potential ecological risk index (RI) grades. Ecological risk grades *(Ei)* are as follows < 40 – Low, 40 to 80 – Moderate, 80 to 160 – Considerable, 160 to 320 – High and ≥ 320 - Very high. Potential ecological risk index (RI) grades are as follows < 150 to Low, 150 to 300 – Moderate, 300 to 600 – Considerable and ≥ 600 – High.

The level of potential ecological risk ranges from 44.96 to 126.42 in Kadinamkulam estuary with a mean value of 104.59 (Table.5.6, Fig. 5.35); 65.53 to 165.78 in Anchuthengu estuary with a mean value of 108.48 (Table.5.8, Fig. 5.35); 93.1 to 272.71 with an average of 143.43 in Kappil – Hariharapuram estuary (Table.5.10, Fig. 5.35) and 86.80 to 211.96 with an average of 112.62 in Kayamkulam estuary (Table.5.12, Fig. 5.35). The grades of ecological risk of the metals suggest that all the elements fall under the low-risk category in Kadinamkulam estuary, 3 samples falling under moderately risk and all remaining samples under low-risk category in Anchuthengu estuary; 7 samples falling under moderately risk and all other samples under low-risk category in Kappil – Hariharapuram estuary and 2 samples falling under moderately risk and all other samples under low-risk category in Kayamkulam estuary.

**Table. 5.5** Enrichment Factor (EF) and Contamination Factor (CF) in the surface sediments, Kadinamkulam estuary, Kerala, India

| S. no | ENRICHMENT FACTOR | | | | | | | CONTAMINATION FACTOR | | | | | | | |
|---|---|---|---|---|---|---|---|---|---|---|---|---|---|---|---|
| | EF Mn | EF Cu | EF Cr | EF Ni | EF Pb | EF Zn | EF Co | CF Fe | CF Mn | CF Cu | CF Cr | CF Ni | CF Pb | CF Zn | CF Co |
| 1 | 3.49 | 13.08 | 18.72 | 6.17 | 5.99 | 6.36 | 1.45 | 0.71 | 2.47 | 9.26 | 13.25 | 4.36 | 4.23 | 4.50 | 1.03 |
| 2 | 4.19 | 12.28 | 17.40 | 6.05 | 10.99 | 10.06 | 2.05 | 0.50 | 2.09 | 6.13 | 8.69 | 3.02 | 5.49 | 5.02 | 1.03 |
| 3 | 17.44 | 0.29 | 0.54 | 0.50 | 3.22 | 0.34 | 0.03 | 1.16 | 20.17 | 0.34 | 0.63 | 0.57 | 3.72 | 0.40 | 0.03 |
| 4 | 4.65 | 2.10 | 10.52 | 3.08 | 6.37 | 6.20 | 1.08 | 1.04 | 4.86 | 2.20 | 10.98 | 3.21 | 6.65 | 6.47 | 1.13 |
| 5 | 4.08 | 4.11 | 12.44 | 3.85 | 8.13 | 6.79 | 1.46 | 0.76 | 3.10 | 3.12 | 9.45 | 2.92 | 6.17 | 5.16 | 1.11 |
| 6 | 7.91 | 2.77 | 8.98 | 2.24 | 5.12 | 3.24 | 0.77 | 1.52 | 12.02 | 4.21 | 13.64 | 3.40 | 7.78 | 4.92 | 1.17 |
| 7 | 3.89 | 6.00 | 9.91 | 2.51 | 5.58 | 4.35 | 0.87 | 1.26 | 4.91 | 7.59 | 12.53 | 3.17 | 7.05 | 5.49 | 1.10 |
| 8 | 3.09 | 1.85 | 9.02 | 2.08 | 4.25 | 2.42 | 0.69 | 1.66 | 5.11 | 3.07 | 14.94 | 3.45 | 7.05 | 4.01 | 1.14 |
| 9 | 3.81 | 1.21 | 9.34 | 1.95 | 4.21 | 1.56 | 0.57 | 1.60 | 6.09 | 1.93 | 14.94 | 3.13 | 6.73 | 2.49 | 0.92 |
| 10 | 5.00 | 2.12 | 9.27 | 2.09 | 4.92 | 2.24 | 0.59 | 1.49 | 7.46 | 3.17 | 13.84 | 3.11 | 7.35 | 3.35 | 0.88 |
| 11 | 3.82 | 1.25 | 12.18 | 2.38 | 4.75 | 1.80 | 0.68 | 1.71 | 6.53 | 2.14 | 20.85 | 4.07 | 8.13 | 3.08 | 1.17 |
| 12 | 2.48 | 1.53 | 8.14 | 1.52 | 3.96 | 1.48 | 0.63 | 1.80 | 4.48 | 2.76 | 14.69 | 2.74 | 7.14 | 2.66 | 1.13 |
| 13 | 3.47 | 1.88 | 7.92 | 1.90 | 4.72 | 1.67 | 0.66 | 1.56 | 5.43 | 2.93 | 12.37 | 2.96 | 7.38 | 2.61 | 1.04 |
| 14 | 3.81 | 1.64 | 16.05 | 4.26 | 7.44 | 2.44 | 1.04 | 0.89 | 3.39 | 1.46 | 14.29 | 3.80 | 6.63 | 2.17 | 0.92 |
| 15 | 1.65 | 2.36 | 9.50 | 2.17 | 4.36 | 3.54 | 0.63 | 1.49 | 2.45 | 3.51 | 14.14 | 3.22 | 6.49 | 5.27 | 0.94 |
| 16 | 3.77 | 1.17 | 10.73 | 2.63 | 4.31 | 1.87 | 0.62 | 1.51 | 5.68 | 1.76 | 16.17 | 3.96 | 6.50 | 2.81 | 0.94 |
| 17 | 2.93 | 2.28 | 7.71 | 1.73 | 3.65 | 2.50 | 0.58 | 2.04 | 6.00 | 4.65 | 15.76 | 3.53 | 7.46 | 5.11 | 1.18 |
| 18 | 3.51 | 4.32 | 11.36 | 2.47 | 5.22 | 2.41 | 0.79 | 1.32 | 4.63 | 5.70 | 14.98 | 3.25 | 6.88 | 3.17 | 1.04 |
| 19 | 3.66 | 1.86 | 11.06 | 2.65 | 7.65 | 2.61 | 1.11 | 0.86 | 3.14 | 1.59 | 9.49 | 2.27 | 6.56 | 2.23 | 0.95 |
| 20 | 3.78 | 6.39 | 10.70 | 2.80 | 5.73 | 4.64 | 0.85 | 1.12 | 4.22 | 7.13 | 11.94 | 3.13 | 6.39 | 5.18 | 0.95 |
| 21 | 3.70 | 4.15 | 13.24 | 3.02 | 7.79 | 3.95 | 0.88 | 1.02 | 3.77 | 4.22 | 13.48 | 3.08 | 7.94 | 4.02 | 0.90 |
| 22 | 3.45 | 2.48 | 9.98 | 2.36 | 5.75 | 2.39 | 0.87 | 1.45 | 5.00 | 3.60 | 14.46 | 3.41 | 8.33 | 3.46 | 1.26 |
| 23 | 3.13 | 3.13 | 15.03 | 3.72 | 5.89 | 2.65 | 0.94 | 1.27 | 3.98 | 3.98 | 19.08 | 4.72 | 7.48 | 3.37 | 1.20 |
| Avg | 4.38 | 3.49 | 10.86 | 2.79 | 5.65 | 3.37 | 0.86 | 1.29 | 5.52 | 3.76 | 13.24 | 3.24 | 6.76 | 3.78 | 1.01 |
| Max | 17.44 | 13.08 | 18.72 | 6.17 | 10.99 | 10.06 | 2.05 | 2.04 | 20.17 | 9.26 | 20.85 | 4.72 | 8.33 | 6.47 | 1.26 |
| Min | 1.65 | 0.29 | 0.54 | 0.50 | 3.22 | 0.34 | 0.03 | 0.50 | 2.09 | 0.34 | 0.63 | 0.57 | 3.72 | 0.40 | 0.03 |

**Table. 5.6** Geo-accumulation index (Igeo) and Pollution indices in the surface sediments, Kadinamkulam estuary, Kerala, India

| S. no | GEO ACCUMULATION INDEX | | | | | | | | POLLUTION INDICES | | |
|---|---|---|---|---|---|---|---|---|---|---|---|
| | Igeo Fe | Igeo Mn | Igeo Cu | Igeo Cr | Igeo Ni | Igeo Pb | Igeo Zn | Igeo Co | PLI | SPI | PERI |
| 1 | -1.08 | 0.72 | 2.63 | 3.14 | 1.54 | 1.50 | 1.58 | -0.55 | 4.05 | 6.01 | 122.74 |
| 2 | -1.59 | 0.48 | 2.03 | 2.53 | 1.01 | 1.87 | 1.74 | -0.55 | 3.34 | 5.40 | 97.69 |
| 3 | -0.38 | 3.75 | -2.15 | -1.26 | -1.39 | 1.31 | -1.92 | -5.56 | 1.23 | 1.95 | 44.96 |
| 4 | -0.52 | 1.69 | 0.55 | 2.87 | 1.10 | 2.15 | 2.11 | -0.41 | 4.02 | 5.59 | 93.58 |
| 5 | -0.98 | 1.05 | 1.06 | 2.65 | 0.96 | 2.04 | 1.78 | -0.44 | 3.50 | 5.23 | 88.23 |
| 6 | 0.02 | 3.00 | 1.49 | 3.19 | 1.18 | 2.38 | 1.71 | -0.36 | 5.42 | 6.61 | 121.22 |
| 7 | -0.25 | 1.71 | 2.34 | 3.06 | 1.08 | 2.23 | 1.87 | -0.44 | 4.95 | 6.80 | 124.50 |
| 8 | 0.14 | 1.77 | 1.03 | 3.32 | 1.20 | 2.23 | 1.42 | -0.39 | 4.51 | 6.11 | 106.85 |
| 9 | 0.09 | 2.02 | 0.36 | 3.32 | 1.06 | 2.17 | 0.73 | -0.71 | 3.94 | 5.56 | 97.40 |
| 10 | -0.01 | 2.31 | 1.08 | 3.21 | 1.05 | 2.29 | 1.16 | -0.77 | 4.50 | 6.05 | 106.67 |
| 11 | 0.19 | 2.12 | 0.51 | 3.80 | 1.44 | 2.44 | 1.04 | -0.36 | 4.70 | 7.00 | 122.99 |
| 12 | 0.27 | 1.58 | 0.88 | 3.29 | 0.87 | 2.25 | 0.83 | -0.41 | 4.02 | 5.82 | 99.74 |
| 13 | 0.06 | 1.85 | 0.97 | 3.04 | 0.98 | 2.30 | 0.80 | -0.53 | 4.04 | 5.79 | 99.17 |
| 14 | -0.75 | 1.18 | -0.04 | 3.25 | 1.34 | 2.14 | 0.54 | -0.70 | 3.20 | 5.47 | 93.59 |
| 15 | -0.01 | 0.71 | 1.23 | 3.24 | 1.10 | 2.11 | 1.81 | -0.67 | 4.11 | 5.94 | 102.10 |
| 16 | 0.01 | 1.92 | 0.23 | 3.43 | 1.40 | 2.12 | 0.91 | -0.68 | 4.04 | 5.72 | 101.92 |
| 17 | 0.45 | 2.00 | 1.63 | 3.39 | 1.23 | 2.31 | 1.77 | -0.35 | 5.32 | 6.78 | 120.84 |
| 18 | -0.19 | 1.63 | 1.93 | 3.32 | 1.12 | 2.20 | 1.08 | -0.53 | 4.49 | 6.40 | 116.93 |
| 19 | -0.81 | 1.07 | 0.09 | 2.66 | 0.60 | 2.13 | 0.58 | -0.66 | 2.80 | 4.75 | 76.48 |
| 20 | -0.43 | 1.49 | 2.25 | 2.99 | 1.06 | 2.09 | 1.79 | -0.66 | 4.57 | 6.33 | 116.54 |
| 21 | -0.56 | 1.33 | 1.49 | 3.17 | 1.04 | 2.40 | 1.42 | -0.74 | 4.16 | 6.53 | 110.92 |
| 22 | -0.05 | 1.74 | 1.26 | 3.27 | 1.19 | 2.47 | 1.20 | -0.26 | 4.49 | 6.69 | 114.09 |
| 23 | -0.24 | 1.41 | 1.41 | 3.67 | 1.65 | 2.32 | 1.17 | -0.33 | 4.63 | 7.02 | 126.42 |
| **Avg** | **-0.29** | **1.68** | **1.05** | **2.98** | **1.04** | **2.15** | **1.18** | **-0.74** | **4.09** | **5.89** | **104.59** |
| **Max** | **0.45** | **3.75** | **2.63** | **3.80** | **1.65** | **2.47** | **2.11** | **-0.26** | **5.42** | **7.02** | **126.42** |
| **Min** | **-1.59** | **0.48** | **-2.15** | **-1.26** | **-1.39** | **1.31** | **-1.92** | **-5.56** | **1.23** | **1.95** | **44.96** |

**Table. 5.7** Enrichment Factor (EF) and Contamination Factor (CF) in the surface sediments, Anchuthengu estuary, Kerala, India

| S.no | ENRICHMENT FACTOR | | | | | | | CONTAMINATION FACTOR | | | | | | | |
|---|---|---|---|---|---|---|---|---|---|---|---|---|---|---|---|
| | EF Mn | EF Cu | EF Cr | EF Ni | EF Pb | EF Zn | EF Co | CF Fe | CF Mn | CF Cu | CF Cr | CF Ni | CF Pb | CF Zn | CF Co |
| 24 | 3.78 | 1.13 | 7.98 | 1.53 | 2.53 | 1.49 | 0.59 | 1.87 | 7.07 | 2.11 | 14.91 | 2.86 | 4.72 | 2.78 | 1.11 |
| 25 | 2.03 | 2.06 | 5.77 | 1.02 | 1.82 | 1.80 | 0.38 | 2.98 | 6.04 | 6.13 | 17.17 | 3.05 | 5.40 | 5.36 | 1.12 |
| 26 | 1.93 | 3.75 | 5.91 | 1.04 | 2.29 | 1.73 | 0.41 | 2.75 | 5.33 | 10.33 | 16.26 | 2.86 | 6.31 | 4.77 | 1.14 |
| 27 | 2.42 | 0.83 | 6.54 | 1.55 | 2.47 | 1.42 | 0.48 | 2.28 | 5.51 | 1.90 | 14.89 | 3.53 | 5.63 | 3.24 | 1.09 |
| 28 | 5.69 | 1.18 | 10.88 | 2.05 | 4.11 | 1.75 | 0.82 | 1.02 | 5.82 | 1.21 | 11.14 | 2.10 | 4.21 | 1.80 | 0.84 |
| 29 | 1.60 | 1.53 | 8.02 | 1.38 | 2.42 | 1.60 | 0.57 | 1.78 | 2.84 | 2.73 | 14.29 | 2.46 | 4.31 | 2.85 | 1.01 |
| 30 | 3.11 | 0.92 | 10.94 | 2.59 | 3.68 | 1.97 | 1.00 | 1.08 | 3.34 | 0.99 | 11.76 | 2.79 | 3.95 | 2.11 | 1.08 |
| 31 | 4.64 | 5.69 | 30.98 | 10.64 | 3.73 | 3.06 | 1.51 | 0.92 | 4.26 | 5.22 | 28.43 | 9.77 | 3.42 | 2.81 | 1.38 |
| 32 | 3.65 | 1.14 | 12.13 | 4.03 | 4.42 | 2.22 | 1.27 | 0.84 | 3.06 | 0.95 | 10.18 | 3.38 | 3.71 | 1.86 | 1.07 |
| 33 | 5.36 | 8.11 | 9.52 | 2.24 | 4.31 | 3.97 | 1.11 | 0.97 | 5.20 | 7.87 | 9.24 | 2.18 | 4.19 | 3.85 | 1.08 |
| 34 | 3.06 | 4.09 | 14.34 | 3.76 | 5.35 | 4.73 | 1.37 | 0.84 | 2.58 | 3.44 | 12.07 | 3.16 | 4.50 | 3.98 | 1.15 |
| 35 | 4.94 | 6.15 | 8.91 | 1.91 | 5.35 | 3.02 | 0.94 | 1.16 | 5.75 | 7.16 | 10.37 | 2.23 | 6.24 | 3.51 | 1.10 |
| 36 | 1.72 | 1.45 | 11.10 | 2.48 | 3.45 | 2.01 | 0.77 | 1.47 | 2.52 | 2.12 | 16.26 | 3.63 | 5.06 | 2.94 | 1.13 |
| 37 | 0.88 | 1.13 | 7.84 | 1.95 | 3.85 | 1.36 | 0.67 | 1.77 | 1.55 | 2.00 | 13.87 | 3.45 | 6.81 | 2.40 | 1.18 |
| 38 | 2.41 | 1.06 | 12.60 | 3.05 | 5.55 | 1.94 | 1.14 | 1.04 | 2.51 | 1.11 | 13.12 | 3.18 | 5.78 | 2.03 | 1.19 |
| 39 | 4.35 | 6.29 | 10.45 | 2.72 | 5.33 | 4.48 | 1.17 | 1.03 | 4.47 | 6.47 | 10.75 | 2.80 | 5.49 | 4.61 | 1.20 |
| 40 | 3.75 | 3.52 | 7.36 | 1.49 | 3.12 | 2.03 | 0.63 | 1.92 | 7.20 | 6.76 | 14.16 | 2.86 | 6.01 | 3.90 | 1.21 |
| 41 | 2.02 | 1.51 | 11.76 | 2.70 | 4.23 | 2.82 | 0.71 | 1.50 | 3.02 | 2.26 | 17.58 | 4.03 | 6.33 | 4.21 | 1.07 |
| 42 | 2.80 | 1.21 | 8.28 | 1.87 | 3.40 | 1.80 | 0.69 | 1.86 | 5.21 | 2.25 | 15.40 | 3.47 | 6.33 | 3.35 | 1.28 |
| 43 | 4.33 | 8.86 | 10.85 | 2.82 | 5.44 | 5.08 | 1.13 | 1.07 | 4.62 | 9.45 | 11.58 | 3.01 | 5.80 | 5.42 | 1.20 |
| 44 | 0.39 | 0.13 | 1.28 | 0.34 | 0.54 | 0.23 | 0.12 | 10.31 | 4.05 | 1.32 | 13.18 | 3.55 | 5.52 | 2.38 | 1.23 |
| 45 | 0.48 | 0.29 | 2.81 | 0.77 | 1.23 | 0.54 | 0.23 | 4.48 | 2.14 | 1.31 | 12.60 | 3.43 | 5.53 | 2.40 | 1.02 |
| 46 | 4.76 | 3.90 | 8.81 | 2.74 | 5.93 | 2.09 | 0.90 | 1.03 | 4.91 | 4.02 | 9.08 | 2.82 | 6.11 | 2.15 | 0.93 |
| 47 | 3.86 | 2.17 | 8.53 | 2.26 | 4.98 | 2.18 | 0.75 | 1.84 | 7.11 | 3.99 | 15.69 | 4.15 | 9.16 | 4.01 | 1.39 |
| 48 | 16.99 | 1.53 | 10.15 | 2.73 | 6.96 | 2.25 | 0.95 | 1.42 | 24.18 | 2.18 | 14.44 | 3.89 | 9.90 | 3.21 | 1.35 |
| 49 | 5.13 | 4.08 | 6.82 | 1.53 | 3.89 | 2.85 | 0.55 | 2.40 | 12.31 | 9.79 | 16.36 | 3.66 | 9.33 | 6.84 | 1.31 |
| 50 | 4.72 | 3.13 | 8.76 | 1.93 | 4.51 | 3.00 | 0.66 | 2.17 | 10.25 | 6.80 | 19.05 | 4.20 | 9.81 | 6.52 | 1.43 |
| 51 | 4.66 | 1.27 | 7.50 | 1.71 | 5.37 | 1.87 | 0.74 | 1.89 | 8.81 | 2.39 | 14.17 | 3.23 | 10.15 | 3.53 | 1.41 |
| 52 | 4.52 | 2.59 | 6.12 | 1.49 | 3.85 | 1.55 | 0.54 | 2.29 | 10.37 | 5.93 | 14.05 | 3.41 | 8.82 | 3.55 | 1.25 |
| 53 | 4.07 | 1.62 | 6.61 | 1.55 | 4.03 | 1.67 | 0.57 | 2.38 | 9.68 | 3.85 | 15.72 | 3.69 | 9.58 | 3.98 | 1.35 |
| 54 | 8.94 | 1.58 | 10.71 | 2.60 | 6.95 | 2.42 | 0.92 | 1.39 | 12.44 | 2.20 | 14.90 | 3.62 | 9.66 | 3.37 | 1.29 |
| 55 | 3.85 | 1.03 | 6.88 | 1.69 | 4.32 | 1.48 | 0.62 | 2.39 | 9.19 | 2.45 | 16.43 | 4.03 | 10.31 | 3.54 | 1.47 |
| Avg | 3.96 | 2.65 | 9.28 | 2.32 | 4.04 | 2.26 | 0.78 | 2.00 | 6.35 | 4.02 | 14.35 | 3.45 | 6.50 | 3.54 | 1.19 |
| Max | 16.99 | 8.86 | 30.98 | 10.64 | 6.96 | 5.08 | 1.51 | 10.31 | 24.18 | 10.33 | 28.43 | 9.77 | 10.31 | 6.84 | 1.47 |
| Min | 0.39 | 0.13 | 1.28 | 0.34 | 0.54 | 0.23 | 0.12 | 0.84 | 1.55 | 0.95 | 9.08 | 2.10 | 3.42 | 1.80 | 0.84 |

**Table. 5.8** Geo-accumulation index (Igeo) and Pollution indices in the surface sediments, Anchuthengu estuary, Kerala, India

| S. no | GEO ACCUMULATION INDEX | | | | | | | | POLLUTION INDICES | | |
|---|---|---|---|---|---|---|---|---|---|---|---|
| | Igeo Fe | Igeo Mn | Igeo Cu | Igeo Cr | Igeo Ni | Igeo Pb | Igeo Zn | Igeo Co | PLI | SPI | PERI |
| 24 | 0.32 | 2.24 | 0.49 | 3.31 | 0.93 | 1.65 | 0.89 | -0.44 | 3.97 | 4.66 | 88.09 |
| 25 | 0.99 | 2.01 | 2.03 | 3.52 | 1.02 | 1.85 | 1.84 | -0.42 | 5.57 | 6.17 | 118.65 |
| 26 | 0.88 | 1.83 | 2.78 | 3.44 | 0.93 | 2.07 | 1.67 | -0.39 | 5.77 | 7.18 | 140.10 |
| 27 | 0.60 | 1.88 | 0.34 | 3.31 | 1.23 | 1.91 | 1.11 | -0.46 | 4.19 | 5.19 | 93.81 |
| 28 | -0.55 | 1.96 | -0.31 | 2.89 | 0.49 | 1.49 | 0.26 | -0.83 | 2.78 | 3.69 | 67.50 |
| 29 | 0.25 | 0.92 | 0.86 | 3.25 | 0.71 | 1.52 | 0.93 | -0.57 | 3.46 | 4.46 | 81.81 |
| 30 | -0.48 | 1.16 | -0.60 | 2.97 | 0.90 | 1.40 | 0.49 | -0.48 | 2.67 | 3.75 | 67.64 |
| 31 | -0.71 | 1.51 | 1.80 | 4.24 | 2.70 | 1.19 | 0.91 | -0.12 | 4.75 | 7.12 | 156.00 |
| 32 | -0.84 | 1.03 | -0.65 | 2.76 | 1.17 | 1.31 | 0.31 | -0.49 | 2.48 | 3.57 | 65.53 |
| 33 | -0.63 | 1.79 | 2.39 | 2.62 | 0.54 | 1.48 | 1.36 | -0.47 | 3.86 | 4.92 | 98.69 |
| 34 | -0.83 | 0.78 | 1.20 | 3.01 | 1.08 | 1.59 | 1.41 | -0.38 | 3.39 | 4.71 | 86.23 |
| 35 | -0.36 | 1.94 | 2.26 | 2.79 | 0.57 | 2.06 | 1.23 | -0.45 | 4.23 | 5.80 | 108.15 |
| 36 | -0.03 | 0.75 | 0.50 | 3.44 | 1.28 | 1.75 | 0.97 | -0.41 | 3.53 | 5.09 | 92.01 |
| 37 | 0.24 | 0.05 | 0.42 | 3.21 | 1.20 | 2.18 | 0.68 | -0.35 | 3.30 | 5.57 | 93.05 |
| 38 | -0.53 | 0.75 | -0.44 | 3.13 | 1.08 | 1.95 | 0.43 | -0.34 | 2.82 | 4.79 | 81.14 |
| 39 | -0.54 | 1.58 | 2.11 | 2.84 | 0.90 | 1.87 | 1.62 | -0.32 | 4.19 | 5.58 | 104.41 |
| 40 | 0.36 | 2.26 | 2.17 | 3.24 | 0.93 | 2.00 | 1.38 | -0.31 | 5.09 | 6.12 | 117.60 |
| 41 | 0.00 | 1.01 | 0.59 | 3.55 | 1.43 | 2.08 | 1.49 | -0.49 | 4.10 | 6.00 | 105.53 |
| 42 | 0.31 | 1.80 | 0.59 | 3.36 | 1.21 | 2.08 | 1.16 | -0.22 | 4.24 | 5.62 | 99.58 |
| 43 | -0.49 | 1.62 | 2.66 | 2.95 | 1.01 | 1.95 | 1.85 | -0.32 | 4.71 | 6.45 | 124.53 |
| 44 | 2.78 | 1.43 | -0.18 | 3.13 | 1.24 | 1.88 | 0.67 | -0.29 | 4.44 | 4.81 | 84.76 |
| 45 | 1.58 | 0.51 | -0.19 | 3.07 | 1.19 | 1.88 | 0.68 | -0.56 | 3.56 | 4.74 | 81.09 |
| 46 | -0.54 | 1.71 | 1.42 | 2.60 | 0.91 | 2.03 | 0.52 | -0.69 | 3.53 | 5.05 | 90.02 |
| 47 | 0.30 | 2.24 | 1.41 | 3.39 | 1.47 | 2.61 | 1.42 | -0.11 | 5.35 | 7.44 | 129.05 |
| 48 | -0.08 | 4.01 | 0.54 | 3.27 | 1.37 | 2.72 | 1.10 | -0.15 | 5.40 | 7.21 | 136.10 |
| 49 | 0.68 | 3.04 | 2.71 | 3.45 | 1.29 | 2.64 | 2.19 | -0.20 | 7.30 | 8.80 | 165.78 |
| 50 | 0.54 | 2.77 | 2.18 | 3.67 | 1.49 | 2.71 | 2.12 | -0.06 | 6.94 | 8.78 | 158.95 |
| 51 | 0.33 | 2.55 | 0.67 | 3.24 | 1.11 | 2.76 | 1.24 | -0.09 | 4.87 | 7.25 | 119.56 |
| 52 | 0.61 | 2.79 | 1.98 | 3.23 | 1.18 | 2.56 | 1.24 | -0.26 | 5.77 | 7.31 | 132.83 |
| 53 | 0.66 | 2.69 | 1.36 | 3.39 | 1.30 | 2.68 | 1.41 | -0.15 | 5.70 | 7.52 | 130.67 |
| 54 | -0.11 | 3.05 | 0.55 | 3.31 | 1.27 | 2.69 | 1.17 | -0.22 | 4.89 | 7.11 | 123.03 |
| 55 | 0.67 | 2.62 | 0.71 | 3.45 | 1.42 | 2.78 | 1.24 | -0.03 | 5.38 | 7.68 | 129.49 |
| **Avg** | **0.17** | **1.82** | **1.07** | **3.22** | **1.14** | **2.04** | **1.16** | **-0.35** | **4.45** | **5.94** | **108.48** |
| **Max** | **2.78** | **4.01** | **2.78** | **4.24** | **2.70** | **2.78** | **2.19** | **-0.03** | **7.30** | **8.80** | **165.78** |
| **Min** | **-0.84** | **0.05** | **-0.65** | **2.60** | **0.49** | **1.19** | **0.26** | **-0.83** | **2.48** | **3.57** | **65.53** |

**Table. 5.9** Enrichment Factor (EF) and Contamination Factor (CF) in the surface sediments, Kappil - Hariharapuram estuary, Kerala, India

| S. no | ENRICHMENT FACTOR | | | | | | | CONTAMINATION FACTOR | | | | | | | |
|---|---|---|---|---|---|---|---|---|---|---|---|---|---|---|---|
| | EF Mn | EF Cu | EF Cr | EF Ni | EF Pb | EF Zn | EF Co | CF Fe | CF Mn | CF Cu | CF Cr | CF Ni | CF Pb | CF Zn | CF Co |
| 56 | 6.42 | 2.66 | 11.10 | 2.76 | 5.66 | 1.88 | 0.71 | 1.48 | 9.49 | 3.93 | 16.40 | 4.08 | 8.37 | 2.78 | 1.05 |
| 57 | 3.93 | 2.57 | 8.10 | 2.11 | 4.72 | 1.81 | 0.68 | 1.87 | 7.36 | 4.81 | 15.14 | 3.94 | 8.82 | 3.39 | 1.27 |
| 58 | 4.06 | 0.91 | 6.43 | 1.56 | 3.45 | 1.01 | 0.54 | 2.55 | 10.34 | 2.32 | 16.37 | 3.97 | 8.79 | 2.58 | 1.37 |
| 59 | 2.78 | 0.92 | 7.10 | 1.59 | 4.09 | 1.94 | 0.46 | 2.34 | 6.51 | 2.16 | 16.58 | 3.70 | 9.56 | 4.54 | 1.08 |
| 60 | 2.97 | 6.37 | 12.21 | 3.17 | 5.87 | 2.67 | 0.79 | 1.47 | 4.36 | 9.35 | 17.92 | 4.65 | 8.62 | 3.92 | 1.15 |
| 61 | 3.03 | 2.74 | 10.09 | 2.72 | 5.24 | 2.66 | 0.63 | 1.71 | 5.19 | 4.68 | 17.25 | 4.65 | 8.96 | 4.55 | 1.08 |
| 62 | 10.33 | 4.44 | 8.87 | 2.14 | 5.42 | 3.58 | 0.60 | 1.69 | 17.47 | 7.50 | 15.01 | 3.63 | 9.17 | 6.05 | 1.01 |
| 63 | 2.78 | 3.08 | 6.45 | 1.31 | 3.02 | 2.51 | 0.44 | 3.09 | 8.60 | 9.50 | 19.91 | 4.04 | 9.32 | 7.76 | 1.35 |
| 64 | 6.87 | 1.49 | 11.06 | 2.67 | 6.28 | 2.18 | 0.84 | 1.34 | 9.21 | 1.99 | 14.83 | 3.58 | 8.41 | 2.93 | 1.12 |
| 65 | 4.63 | 2.43 | 7.82 | 1.86 | 4.30 | 2.24 | 0.57 | 2.04 | 9.44 | 4.97 | 15.96 | 3.79 | 8.78 | 4.57 | 1.17 |
| 66 | 1.75 | 2.79 | 7.99 | 2.00 | 4.04 | 1.89 | 0.52 | 1.99 | 3.49 | 5.55 | 15.90 | 3.97 | 8.03 | 3.75 | 1.04 |
| 67 | 4.48 | 15.68 | 8.94 | 2.48 | 6.49 | 8.84 | 0.71 | 1.21 | 5.40 | 18.92 | 10.79 | 2.99 | 7.83 | 10.67 | 0.86 |
| 68 | 6.67 | 7.94 | 13.13 | 3.35 | 8.43 | 8.54 | 1.11 | 0.92 | 6.15 | 7.33 | 12.12 | 3.10 | 7.78 | 7.88 | 1.03 |
| 69 | 4.29 | 23.59 | 8.58 | 2.20 | 6.04 | 7.01 | 0.79 | 1.45 | 6.23 | 34.29 | 12.48 | 3.19 | 8.78 | 10.19 | 1.14 |
| 70 | 3.11 | 3.11 | 8.50 | 2.10 | 4.62 | 3.10 | 0.66 | 1.95 | 6.08 | 6.08 | 16.59 | 4.09 | 9.02 | 6.05 | 1.29 |
| 71 | 3.19 | 7.68 | 6.76 | 1.62 | 3.93 | 4.50 | 0.56 | 2.19 | 7.00 | 16.86 | 14.84 | 3.56 | 8.63 | 9.87 | 1.22 |
| 72 | 4.98 | 4.99 | 12.35 | 2.84 | 6.67 | 4.27 | 0.90 | 1.01 | 5.04 | 5.05 | 12.48 | 2.87 | 6.75 | 4.31 | 0.91 |
| 73 | 2.98 | 2.99 | 10.20 | 2.96 | 4.54 | 2.34 | 0.65 | 1.76 | 5.26 | 5.26 | 17.98 | 5.21 | 8.00 | 4.12 | 1.15 |
| 74 | 2.99 | 7.97 | 10.15 | 2.40 | 6.08 | 6.85 | 0.83 | 1.37 | 4.10 | 10.90 | 13.88 | 3.28 | 8.32 | 9.37 | 1.14 |
| 75 | 2.27 | 3.24 | 6.30 | 1.32 | 3.76 | 3.49 | 0.50 | 2.54 | 5.75 | 8.23 | 15.99 | 3.36 | 9.54 | 8.87 | 1.28 |
| 76 | 3.44 | 4.12 | 10.26 | 2.57 | 5.12 | 2.66 | 0.70 | 1.27 | 4.35 | 5.22 | 13.01 | 3.26 | 6.48 | 3.37 | 0.88 |
| 77 | 3.72 | 4.60 | 9.59 | 2.13 | 5.31 | 2.09 | 0.66 | 1.76 | 6.54 | 8.08 | 16.82 | 3.74 | 9.31 | 3.67 | 1.16 |
| 78 | 6.09 | 4.54 | 11.65 | 2.80 | 9.17 | 2.53 | 0.40 | 0.95 | 5.80 | 4.32 | 11.10 | 2.66 | 8.73 | 2.41 | 0.38 |
| 79 | 3.35 | 6.74 | 10.59 | 3.00 | 6.54 | 5.96 | 0.87 | 1.15 | 3.84 | 7.71 | 12.13 | 3.43 | 7.49 | 6.82 | 1.00 |
| 80 | 3.05 | 2.09 | 9.80 | 2.83 | 7.27 | 1.73 | 0.80 | 1.09 | 3.33 | 2.28 | 10.70 | 3.08 | 7.93 | 1.89 | 0.87 |
| 81 | 3.28 | 3.56 | 8.24 | 1.83 | 4.47 | 2.52 | 0.42 | 1.90 | 6.22 | 6.74 | 15.62 | 3.48 | 8.48 | 4.77 | 0.80 |
| 82 | 4.41 | 9.40 | 9.69 | 2.41 | 5.65 | 5.38 | 0.69 | 1.61 | 7.08 | 15.11 | 15.57 | 3.87 | 9.08 | 8.65 | 1.11 |
| Avg | 4.14 | 5.28 | 9.33 | 2.32 | 5.41 | 3.56 | 0.67 | 1.69 | 6.65 | 8.12 | 14.94 | 3.67 | 8.48 | 5.55 | 1.07 |
| Max | 10.33 | 23.59 | 13.13 | 3.35 | 9.17 | 8.84 | 1.11 | 3.09 | 17.47 | 34.29 | 19.91 | 5.21 | 9.56 | 10.67 | 1.37 |
| Min | 1.75 | 0.91 | 6.30 | 1.31 | 3.02 | 1.01 | 0.40 | 0.92 | 3.33 | 1.99 | 10.70 | 2.66 | 6.48 | 1.89 | 0.38 |

**Table. 5.10** Geo-accumulation index (Igeo) and Pollution indices in the surface sediments, Kappil - Hariharapuram estuary, Kerala, India

| S. no | GEO ACCUMULATION INDEX | | | | | | | | POLLUTION INDICES | | |
|---|---|---|---|---|---|---|---|---|---|---|---|
| | Igeo Fe | Igeo Mn | Igeo Cu | Igeo Cr | Igeo Ni | Igeo Pb | Igeo Zn | Igeo Co | PLI | SPI | PERI |
| 56 | -0.02 | 2.66 | 1.39 | 3.45 | 1.44 | 2.48 | 0.89 | -0.51 | 5.07 | 7.00 | 126.99 |
| 57 | 0.32 | 2.29 | 1.68 | 3.34 | 1.39 | 2.56 | 1.18 | -0.24 | 5.30 | 7.28 | 128.87 |
| 58 | 0.76 | 2.78 | 0.63 | 3.45 | 1.40 | 2.55 | 0.78 | -0.13 | 5.10 | 6.86 | 121.06 |
| 59 | 0.64 | 2.12 | 0.52 | 3.47 | 1.30 | 2.67 | 1.60 | -0.48 | 5.08 | 7.33 | 121.30 |
| 60 | -0.03 | 1.54 | 2.64 | 3.58 | 1.63 | 2.52 | 1.39 | -0.38 | 5.58 | 8.45 | 157.17 |
| 61 | 0.19 | 1.79 | 1.64 | 3.52 | 1.63 | 2.58 | 1.60 | -0.48 | 5.41 | 7.75 | 135.67 |
| 62 | 0.17 | 3.54 | 2.32 | 3.32 | 1.27 | 2.61 | 2.01 | -0.57 | 6.79 | 8.10 | 154.99 |
| 63 | 1.04 | 2.52 | 2.66 | 3.73 | 1.43 | 2.63 | 2.37 | -0.15 | 7.60 | 9.21 | 170.46 |
| 64 | -0.16 | 2.62 | 0.41 | 3.31 | 1.25 | 2.49 | 0.97 | -0.42 | 4.40 | 6.45 | 111.72 |
| 65 | 0.44 | 2.65 | 1.73 | 3.41 | 1.34 | 2.55 | 1.61 | -0.36 | 5.84 | 7.45 | 133.58 |
| 66 | 0.41 | 1.22 | 1.89 | 3.41 | 1.40 | 2.42 | 1.32 | -0.53 | 4.95 | 7.17 | 126.78 |
| 67 | -0.31 | 1.85 | 3.66 | 2.85 | 1.00 | 2.38 | 2.83 | -0.80 | 6.15 | 9.49 | 186.36 |
| 68 | -0.70 | 2.04 | 2.29 | 3.01 | 1.05 | 2.38 | 2.39 | -0.55 | 5.15 | 7.25 | 129.31 |
| 69 | -0.05 | 2.06 | 4.51 | 3.06 | 1.09 | 2.55 | 2.76 | -0.39 | 7.30 | 12.87 | 272.71 |
| 70 | 0.38 | 2.02 | 2.02 | 3.47 | 1.45 | 2.59 | 2.01 | -0.22 | 5.96 | 8.01 | 141.23 |
| 71 | 0.55 | 2.22 | 3.49 | 3.31 | 1.25 | 2.53 | 2.72 | -0.29 | 7.36 | 9.88 | 191.81 |
| 72 | -0.57 | 1.75 | 1.75 | 3.06 | 0.94 | 2.17 | 1.52 | -0.72 | 4.29 | 6.03 | 107.65 |
| 73 | 0.23 | 1.81 | 1.81 | 3.58 | 1.80 | 2.41 | 1.46 | -0.38 | 5.49 | 7.55 | 137.67 |
| 74 | -0.13 | 1.45 | 2.86 | 3.21 | 1.13 | 2.47 | 2.64 | -0.39 | 5.79 | 8.47 | 153.74 |
| 75 | 0.76 | 1.94 | 2.46 | 3.41 | 1.16 | 2.67 | 2.56 | -0.23 | 6.60 | 8.70 | 152.25 |
| 76 | -0.24 | 1.54 | 1.80 | 3.12 | 1.12 | 2.11 | 1.17 | -0.76 | 4.29 | 5.98 | 108.58 |
| 77 | 0.23 | 2.12 | 2.43 | 3.49 | 1.32 | 2.63 | 1.29 | -0.37 | 5.72 | 8.25 | 149.53 |
| 78 | -0.65 | 1.95 | 1.53 | 2.89 | 0.83 | 2.54 | 0.68 | -1.98 | 3.94 | 6.47 | 109.00 |
| 79 | -0.39 | 1.36 | 2.36 | 3.02 | 1.19 | 2.32 | 2.19 | -0.58 | 4.94 | 7.16 | 128.12 |
| 80 | -0.46 | 1.15 | 0.60 | 2.83 | 1.04 | 2.40 | 0.33 | -0.79 | 3.28 | 5.73 | 93.10 |
| 81 | 0.34 | 2.05 | 2.17 | 3.38 | 1.21 | 2.50 | 1.67 | -0.91 | 5.61 | 7.57 | 135.73 |
| 82 | 0.10 | 2.24 | 3.33 | 3.38 | 1.37 | 2.60 | 2.53 | -0.43 | 6.99 | 9.78 | 187.19 |
| **Avg** | **0.11** | **2.05** | **2.10** | **3.30** | **1.28** | **2.49** | **1.72** | **-0.52** | **5.56** | **7.86** | **143.43** |
| **Max** | **1.04** | **3.54** | **4.51** | **3.73** | **1.80** | **2.67** | **2.83** | **-0.13** | **7.60** | **12.87** | **272.71** |
| **Min** | **-0.70** | **1.15** | **0.41** | **2.83** | **0.83** | **2.11** | **0.33** | **-1.98** | **3.28** | **5.73** | **93.10** |

**Table. 5.11** Enrichment Factor (EF) and Contamination Factor (CF) in the surface sediments, Kayamkulam estuary, Kerala, India

| S. no | ENRICHMENT FACTOR | | | | | | | CONTAMINATION FACTOR | | | | | | | |
|---|---|---|---|---|---|---|---|---|---|---|---|---|---|---|---|
| | EF Mn | EF Cu | EF Cr | EF Ni | EF Pb | EF Zn | EF Co | CF Fe | CF Mn | CF Cu | CF Cr | CF Ni | CF Pb | CF Zn | CF Co |
| 83 | 5.99 | 2.11 | 10.19 | 2.66 | 7.23 | 5.39 | 0.88 | 1.07 | 6.38 | 2.25 | 10.85 | 2.84 | 7.71 | 5.74 | 0.94 |
| 84 | 4.31 | 0.94 | 12.58 | 3.23 | 3.46 | 2.22 | 0.78 | 2.34 | 10.07 | 2.19 | 29.43 | 7.56 | 8.10 | 5.19 | 1.83 |
| 85 | 4.87 | 1.07 | 9.72 | 2.29 | 6.33 | 3.08 | 0.99 | 1.50 | 7.33 | 1.62 | 14.62 | 3.45 | 9.52 | 4.64 | 1.49 |
| 86 | 4.72 | 0.97 | 10.96 | 2.59 | 4.87 | 2.47 | 1.32 | 1.68 | 7.92 | 1.63 | 18.42 | 4.35 | 8.18 | 4.16 | 2.22 |
| 87 | 5.53 | 1.54 | 9.85 | 2.53 | 5.93 | 3.21 | 0.76 | 1.27 | 7.04 | 1.96 | 12.53 | 3.21 | 7.54 | 4.08 | 0.97 |
| 88 | 5.63 | 1.35 | 17.78 | 1.76 | 5.25 | 2.04 | 0.42 | 1.49 | 8.42 | 2.02 | 26.56 | 2.63 | 7.85 | 3.05 | 0.62 |
| 89 | 7.16 | 1.06 | 24.49 | 5.30 | 9.74 | 2.12 | 3.81 | 0.79 | 5.64 | 0.84 | 19.30 | 4.17 | 7.68 | 1.67 | 3.01 |
| 90 | 4.45 | 0.49 | 8.90 | 1.91 | 5.45 | 1.64 | 3.37 | 1.38 | 6.12 | 0.67 | 12.24 | 2.63 | 7.49 | 2.25 | 4.63 |
| 91 | 6.87 | 1.00 | 20.48 | 6.00 | 10.89 | 3.32 | 3.43 | 0.67 | 4.60 | 0.67 | 13.70 | 4.01 | 7.29 | 2.22 | 2.29 |
| 92 | 7.74 | 1.20 | 24.39 | 4.87 | 15.16 | 3.07 | 4.09 | 0.53 | 4.07 | 0.63 | 12.82 | 2.56 | 7.96 | 1.61 | 2.15 |
| 93 | 4.95 | 0.77 | 10.98 | 2.54 | 6.81 | 1.99 | 1.99 | 1.23 | 6.06 | 0.95 | 13.45 | 3.11 | 8.34 | 2.44 | 2.44 |
| 94 | 5.02 | 2.03 | 12.69 | 2.59 | 5.99 | 2.94 | 0.80 | 1.46 | 7.33 | 2.97 | 18.54 | 3.78 | 8.75 | 4.29 | 1.17 |
| 95 | 4.02 | 0.68 | 8.46 | 1.57 | 4.57 | 1.58 | 0.54 | 1.91 | 7.69 | 1.29 | 16.20 | 3.01 | 8.76 | 3.03 | 1.04 |
| 96 | 3.94 | 1.57 | 22.67 | 7.33 | 4.75 | 1.89 | 1.12 | 1.77 | 6.99 | 2.79 | 40.23 | 13.01 | 8.43 | 3.35 | 2.00 |
| 97 | 3.62 | 0.77 | 7.90 | 1.58 | 3.83 | 1.48 | 0.58 | 2.36 | 8.53 | 1.82 | 18.63 | 3.72 | 9.03 | 3.49 | 1.37 |
| 98 | 3.23 | 0.81 | 7.01 | 1.36 | 3.18 | 1.29 | 0.40 | 2.63 | 8.50 | 2.14 | 18.45 | 3.57 | 8.38 | 3.39 | 1.05 |
| 99 | 6.46 | 1.42 | 11.53 | 2.18 | 6.63 | 1.59 | 0.50 | 1.18 | 7.64 | 1.68 | 13.63 | 2.58 | 7.83 | 1.88 | 0.59 |
| 100 | 3.40 | 0.68 | 7.48 | 1.40 | 3.60 | 1.37 | 0.62 | 2.36 | 8.03 | 1.60 | 17.64 | 3.29 | 8.49 | 3.22 | 1.47 |
| 101 | 2.86 | 0.63 | 7.40 | 1.39 | 3.23 | 1.41 | 0.55 | 2.74 | 7.84 | 1.73 | 20.28 | 3.82 | 8.86 | 3.86 | 1.52 |
| 102 | 5.83 | 0.56 | 11.59 | 2.69 | 8.02 | 2.16 | 2.45 | 1.00 | 5.84 | 0.56 | 11.62 | 2.69 | 8.04 | 2.16 | 2.45 |
| 103 | 6.11 | 0.49 | 10.24 | 2.09 | 6.16 | 1.72 | 2.48 | 1.35 | 8.25 | 0.66 | 13.83 | 2.83 | 8.33 | 2.33 | 3.35 |
| 104 | 3.48 | 0.61 | 9.24 | 1.63 | 3.62 | 1.42 | 0.89 | 2.12 | 7.38 | 1.29 | 19.58 | 3.45 | 7.68 | 3.00 | 1.88 |
| 105 | 4.44 | 0.60 | 9.95 | 1.86 | 4.59 | 1.58 | 1.29 | 1.59 | 7.06 | 0.96 | 15.80 | 2.95 | 7.29 | 2.50 | 2.04 |
| 106 | 5.47 | 0.54 | 11.71 | 2.90 | 5.73 | 2.06 | 2.61 | 1.39 | 7.58 | 0.75 | 16.22 | 4.02 | 7.94 | 2.85 | 3.61 |
| 107 | 5.81 | 0.83 | 21.39 | 4.75 | 10.58 | 2.81 | 3.87 | 0.79 | 4.60 | 0.65 | 16.91 | 3.75 | 8.37 | 2.22 | 3.06 |
| 108 | 4.44 | 0.75 | 9.67 | 2.80 | 4.05 | 1.78 | 0.93 | 2.09 | 9.27 | 1.56 | 20.15 | 5.83 | 8.44 | 3.71 | 1.94 |
| 109 | 5.16 | 1.16 | 11.30 | 2.97 | 6.60 | 2.29 | 0.83 | 1.25 | 6.45 | 1.44 | 14.12 | 3.71 | 8.25 | 2.86 | 1.03 |
| 110 | 6.12 | 0.72 | 12.16 | 3.08 | 7.33 | 2.34 | 2.28 | 1.00 | 6.11 | 0.72 | 12.14 | 3.07 | 7.32 | 2.33 | 2.28 |
| 111 | 6.79 | 0.70 | 12.48 | 2.30 | 6.01 | 1.81 | 0.89 | 1.48 | 10.05 | 1.03 | 18.49 | 3.41 | 8.90 | 2.68 | 1.32 |
| Avg | 5.12 | 0.97 | 12.59 | 2.83 | 6.19 | 2.21 | 1.57 | 1.53 | 7.20 | 1.42 | 17.46 | 3.90 | 8.16 | 3.11 | 1.92 |
| Max | 7.74 | 2.11 | 24.49 | 7.33 | 15.16 | 5.39 | 4.09 | 2.74 | 10.07 | 2.97 | 40.23 | 13.01 | 9.52 | 5.74 | 4.63 |
| Min | 2.86 | 0.49 | 7.01 | 1.36 | 3.18 | 1.29 | 0.40 | 0.53 | 4.07 | 0.56 | 10.85 | 2.56 | 7.29 | 1.61 | 0.59 |

**Table. 5.12** Geo-accumulation index (Igeo) and Pollution indices in the surface sediments, Kayamkulam estuary, Kerala, India

| S. no | GEO ACCUMULATION INDEX | | | | | | | | POLLUTION INDICES | | |
|---|---|---|---|---|---|---|---|---|---|---|---|
| | Igeo Fe | Igeo Mn | Igeo Cu | Igeo Cr | Igeo Ni | Igeo Pb | Igeo Zn | Igeo Co | PLI | SPI | PERI |
| 83 | -0.49 | 2.09 | 0.59 | 2.85 | 0.92 | 2.36 | 1.94 | -0.67 | 4.14 | 5.94 | 97.80 |
| 84 | 0.64 | 2.75 | 0.55 | 4.29 | 2.33 | 2.43 | 1.79 | 0.29 | 6.49 | 8.60 | 163.35 |
| 85 | 0.00 | 2.29 | 0.11 | 3.28 | 1.20 | 2.67 | 1.63 | -0.01 | 4.54 | 7.00 | 114.14 |
| 86 | 0.16 | 2.40 | 0.12 | 3.62 | 1.53 | 2.45 | 1.47 | 0.56 | 4.80 | 6.86 | 119.70 |
| 87 | -0.24 | 2.23 | 0.38 | 3.06 | 1.10 | 2.33 | 1.44 | -0.63 | 4.16 | 5.88 | 99.76 |
| 88 | -0.01 | 2.49 | 0.43 | 4.15 | 0.81 | 2.39 | 1.03 | -1.27 | 4.58 | 7.11 | 127.09 |
| 89 | -0.93 | 1.91 | -0.84 | 3.69 | 1.48 | 2.36 | 0.16 | 1.00 | 3.25 | 6.31 | 109.36 |
| 90 | -0.13 | 2.03 | -1.16 | 3.03 | 0.81 | 2.32 | 0.59 | 1.63 | 3.15 | 5.32 | 86.80 |
| 91 | -1.17 | 1.62 | -1.17 | 3.19 | 1.42 | 2.28 | 0.57 | 0.61 | 2.92 | 5.61 | 94.04 |
| 92 | -1.51 | 1.44 | -1.25 | 3.09 | 0.77 | 2.41 | 0.11 | 0.52 | 2.47 | 5.51 | 87.08 |
| 93 | -0.29 | 2.01 | -0.66 | 3.16 | 1.05 | 2.48 | 0.70 | 0.70 | 3.47 | 5.98 | 97.42 |
| 94 | -0.04 | 2.29 | 0.99 | 3.63 | 1.33 | 2.54 | 1.52 | -0.36 | 5.05 | 7.28 | 126.19 |
| 95 | 0.35 | 2.36 | -0.21 | 3.43 | 1.00 | 2.55 | 1.01 | -0.53 | 4.24 | 6.51 | 108.40 |
| 96 | 0.24 | 2.22 | 0.89 | 4.75 | 3.12 | 2.49 | 1.16 | 0.41 | 6.54 | 10.67 | 211.96 |
| 97 | 0.65 | 2.51 | 0.28 | 3.63 | 1.31 | 2.59 | 1.22 | -0.13 | 5.02 | 7.13 | 122.20 |
| 98 | 0.81 | 2.50 | 0.51 | 3.62 | 1.25 | 2.48 | 1.18 | -0.51 | 5.10 | 6.83 | 119.26 |
| 99 | -0.34 | 2.35 | 0.16 | 3.18 | 0.78 | 2.38 | 0.33 | -1.35 | 3.60 | 5.75 | 97.25 |
| 100 | 0.65 | 2.42 | 0.10 | 3.56 | 1.13 | 2.50 | 1.10 | -0.03 | 4.67 | 6.65 | 113.46 |
| 101 | 0.87 | 2.39 | 0.21 | 3.76 | 1.35 | 2.56 | 1.36 | 0.02 | 5.17 | 7.23 | 124.32 |
| 102 | -0.58 | 1.96 | -1.42 | 2.95 | 0.85 | 2.42 | 0.53 | 0.71 | 2.91 | 5.50 | 87.69 |
| 103 | -0.15 | 2.46 | -1.18 | 3.21 | 0.91 | 2.47 | 0.64 | 1.16 | 3.43 | 5.89 | 97.36 |
| 104 | 0.50 | 2.30 | -0.21 | 3.71 | 1.20 | 2.36 | 1.00 | 0.33 | 4.39 | 6.40 | 111.64 |
| 105 | 0.08 | 2.23 | -0.65 | 3.40 | 0.98 | 2.28 | 0.74 | 0.45 | 3.68 | 5.69 | 97.13 |
| 106 | -0.11 | 2.34 | -1.00 | 3.43 | 1.42 | 2.40 | 0.93 | 1.27 | 3.81 | 6.21 | 106.42 |
| 107 | -0.92 | 1.62 | -1.20 | 3.50 | 1.32 | 2.48 | 0.57 | 1.03 | 3.11 | 6.34 | 104.52 |
| 108 | 0.48 | 2.63 | 0.06 | 3.75 | 1.96 | 2.49 | 1.31 | 0.37 | 5.26 | 7.35 | 132.42 |
| 109 | -0.26 | 2.10 | -0.06 | 3.23 | 1.30 | 2.46 | 0.93 | -0.54 | 3.93 | 6.23 | 104.56 |
| 110 | -0.59 | 2.03 | -1.06 | 3.02 | 1.03 | 2.29 | 0.64 | 0.60 | 3.11 | 5.33 | 88.28 |
| 111 | -0.02 | 2.74 | -0.54 | 3.62 | 1.19 | 2.57 | 0.84 | -0.18 | 4.20 | 6.78 | 116.43 |
| **Avg** | **-0.08** | **2.23** | **-0.25** | **3.48** | **1.27** | **2.44** | **0.98** | **0.19** | **4.18** | **6.55** | **112.62** |
| **Max** | **0.87** | **2.75** | **0.99** | **4.75** | **3.12** | **2.67** | **1.94** | **1.63** | **6.54** | **10.67** | **211.96** |
| **Min** | **-1.51** | **1.44** | **-1.42** | **2.85** | **0.77** | **2.28** | **0.11** | **-1.35** | **2.47** | **5.32** | **86.80** |

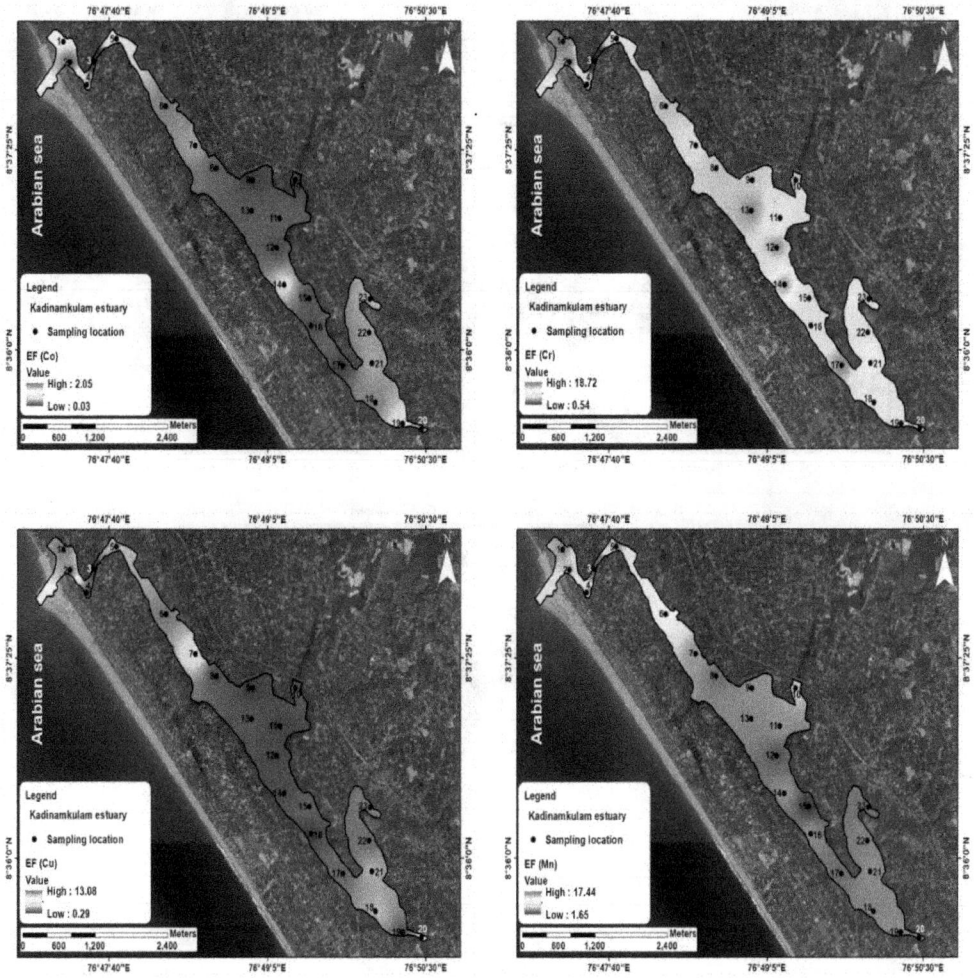

**Fig. 5.9** Spatial distribution map of the Enrichment Factor (EF), in the surface sediments, Kadinamkulam estuary, Kerala, India

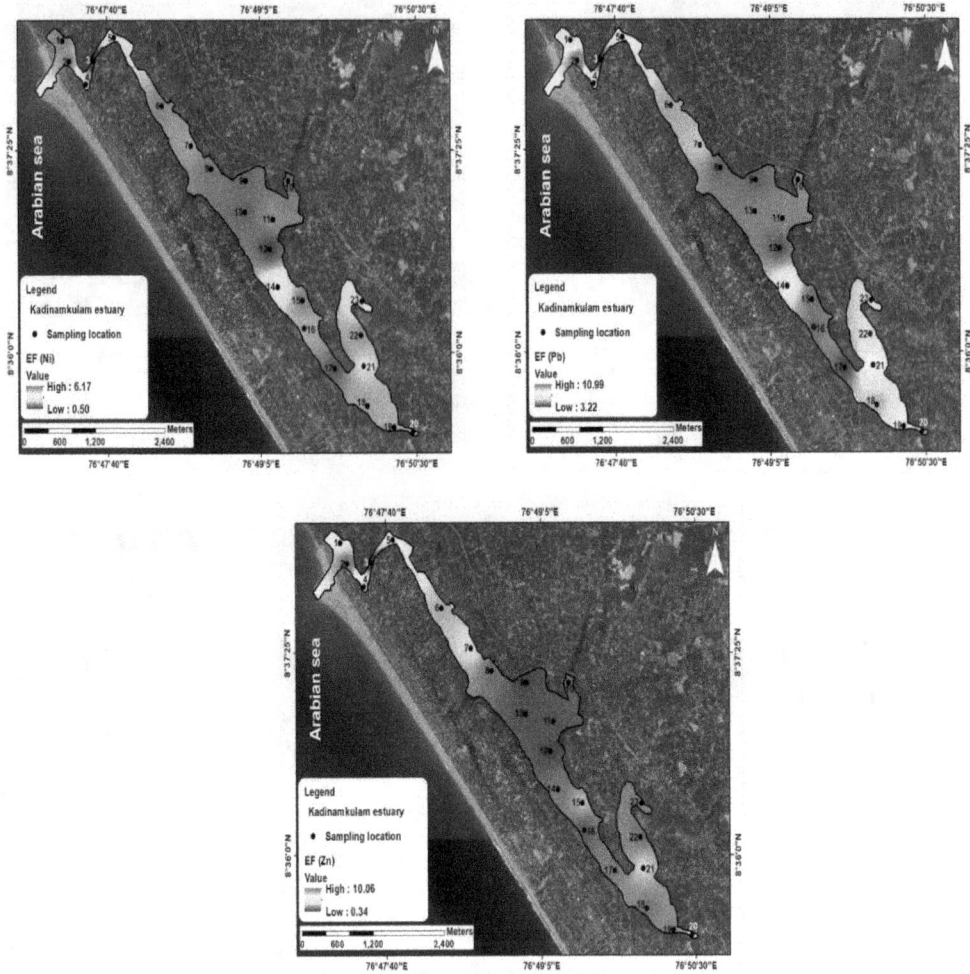

**Fig. 5.10** Spatial distribution map of the Enrichment Factor (EF), in the surface sediments, Kadinamkulam estuary, Kerala, India

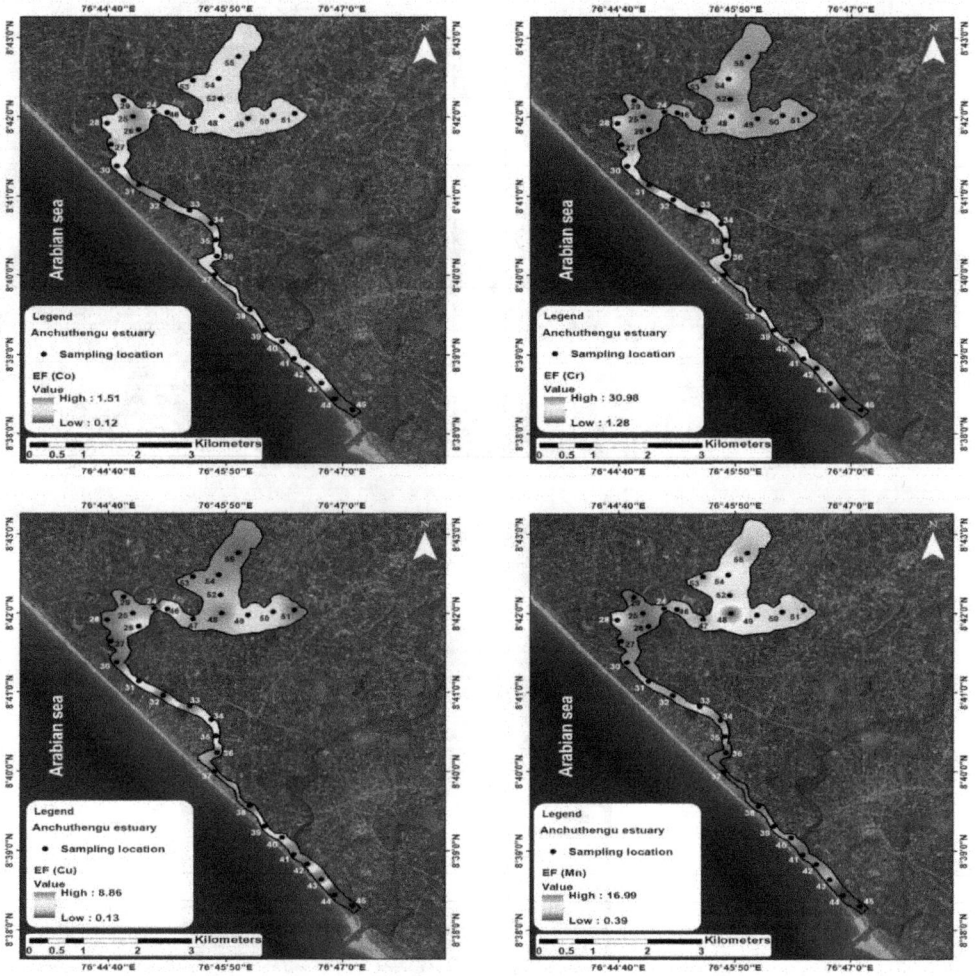

**Fig. 5.11** Spatial distribution map of the Enrichment Factor (EF), in the surface sediments, Anchuthengu estuary, Kerala, India

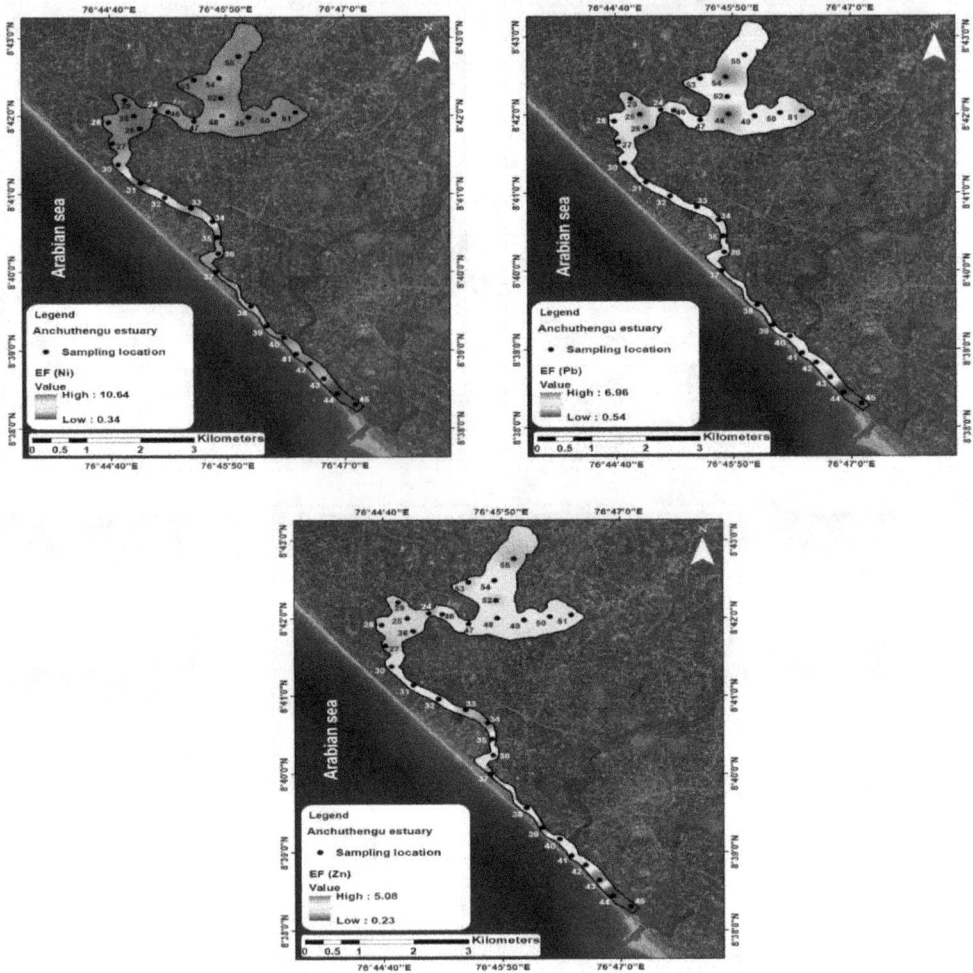

**Fig. 5.12** Spatial distribution map of the Enrichment Factor (EF), in the surface sediments, Anchuthengu estuary, Kerala, India

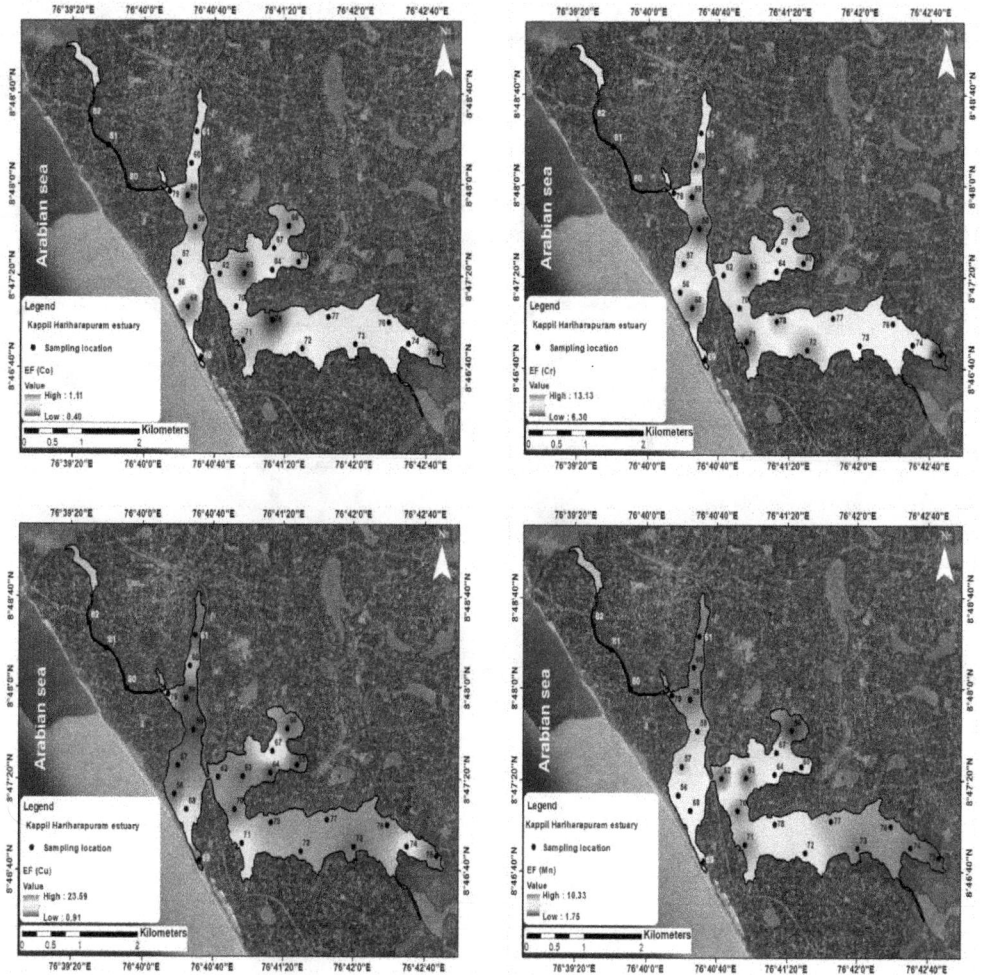

**Fig. 5.13** Spatial distribution map of the Enrichment Factor (EF), in the surface sediments, Kappil - Hariharapuram estuary, Kerala, India

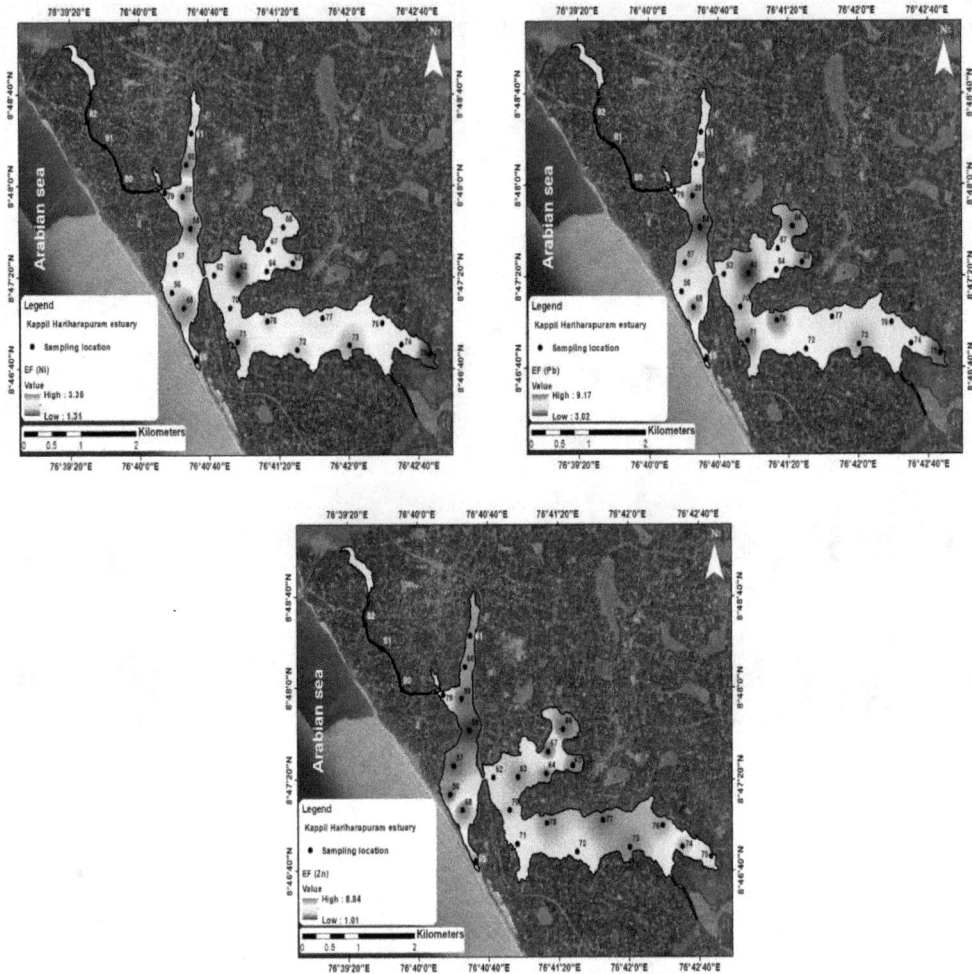

**Fig. 5.14** Spatial distribution map of the Enrichment Factor (EF), in the surface sediments, Kappil - Hariharapuram estuary, Kerala, India

Department of Geology, UNOM

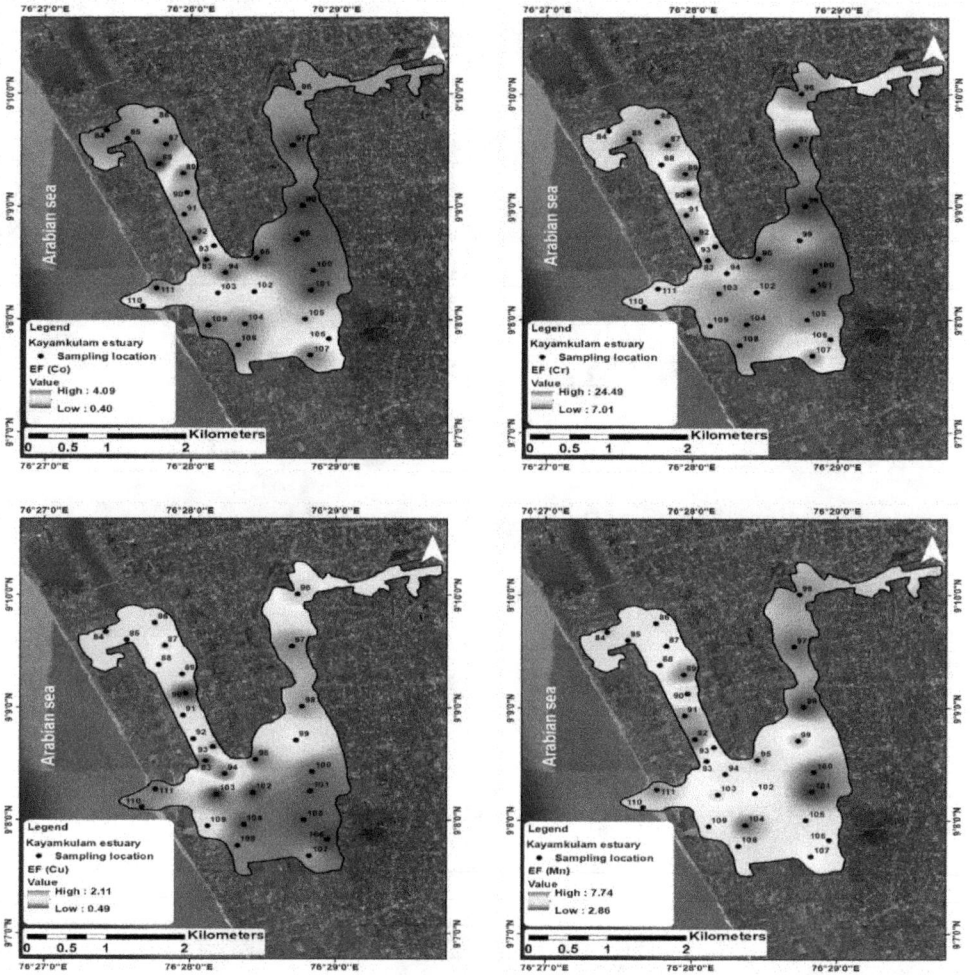

**Fig. 5.15** Spatial distribution map of the Enrichment Factor (EF), in the surface sediments, Kayamkulam estuary, Kerala, India

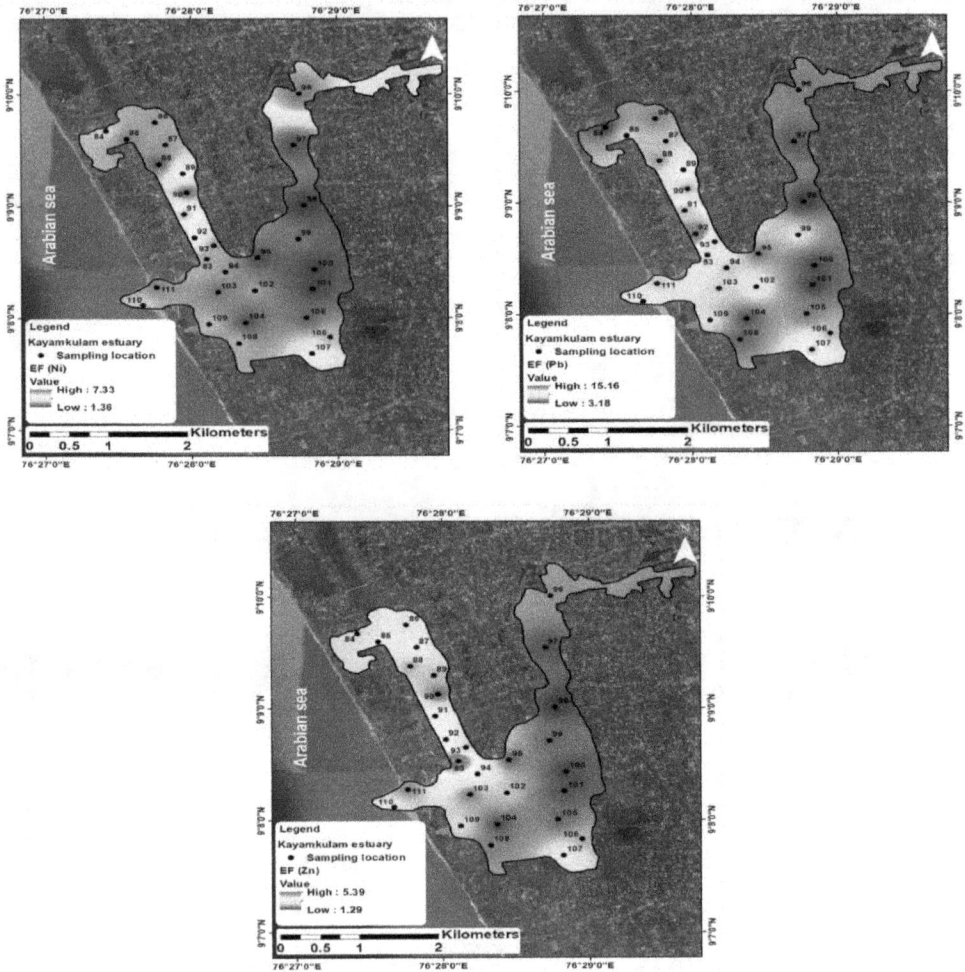

**Fig. 5.16** Spatial distribution map of the Enrichment Factor (EF), in the surface sediments, Kayamkulam estuary, Kerala, India

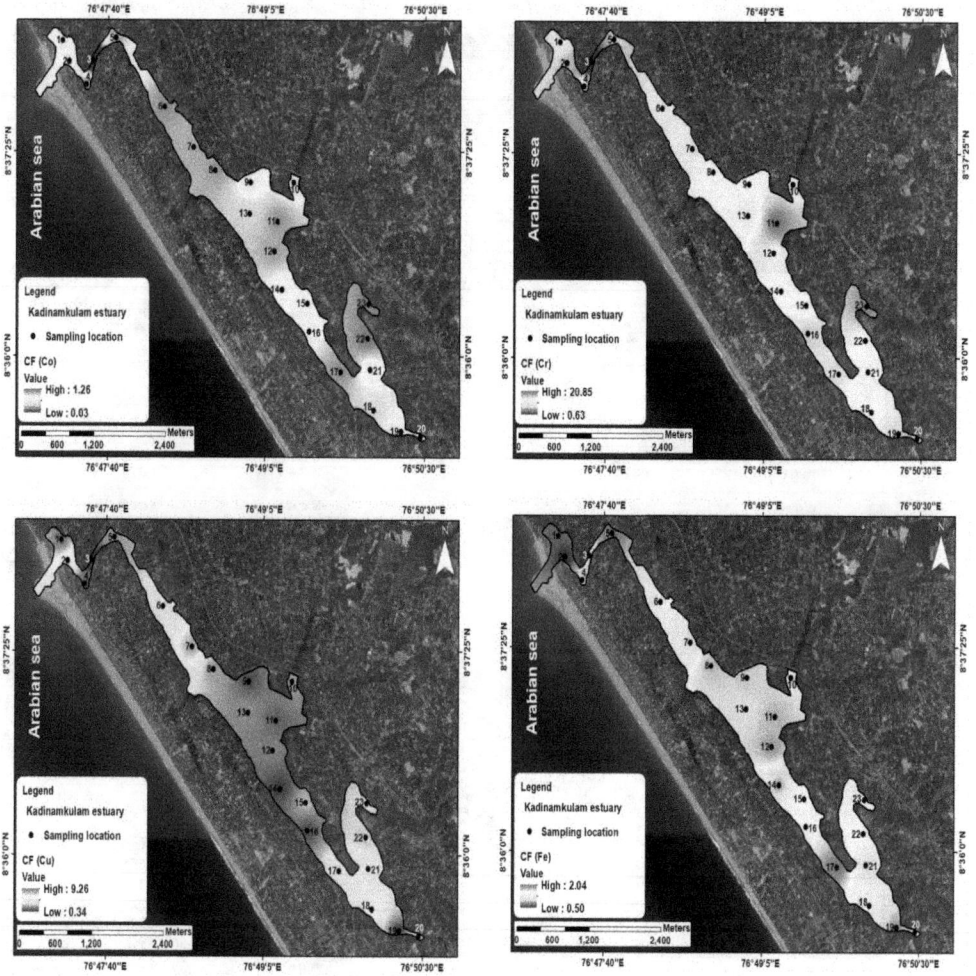

**Fig. 5.17** Spatial distribution map of the Contamination Factor (CF), in the surface sediments, Kadinamkulam estuary, Kerala, India

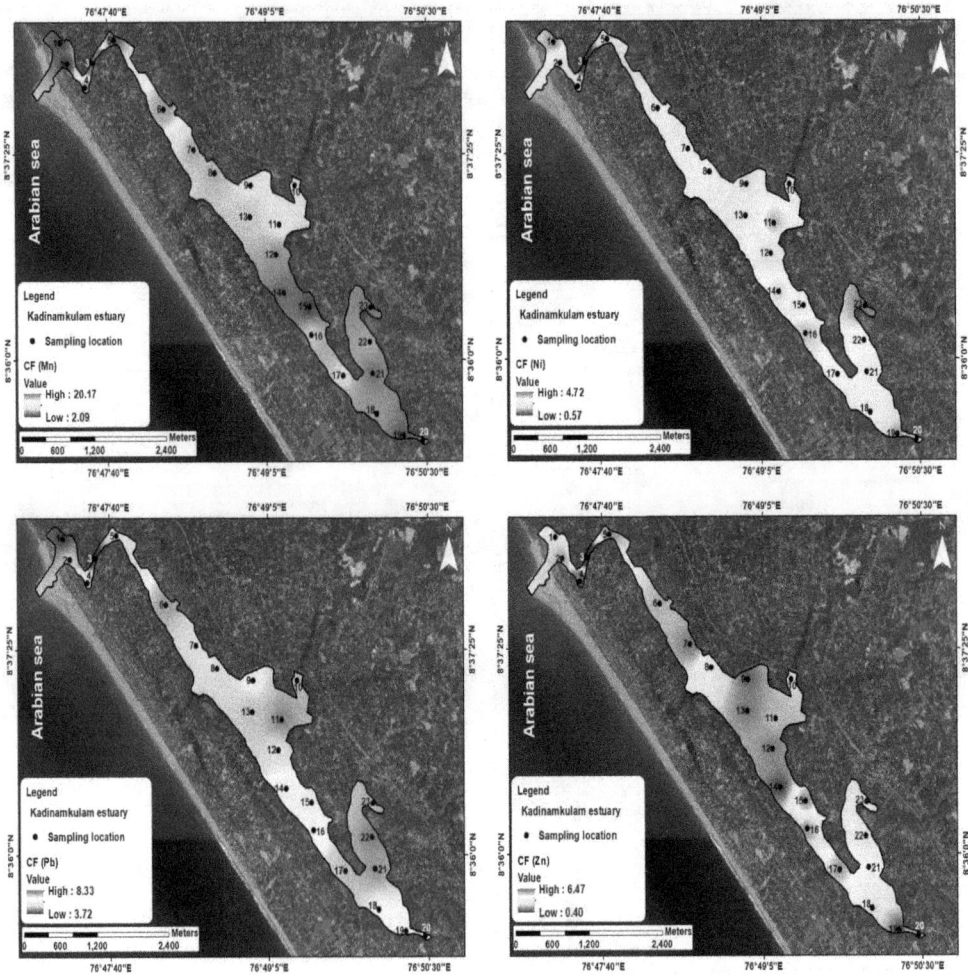

**Fig. 5.18** Spatial distribution map of the Contamination Factor (CF), in the surface sediments, Kadinamkulam estuary, Kerala, India

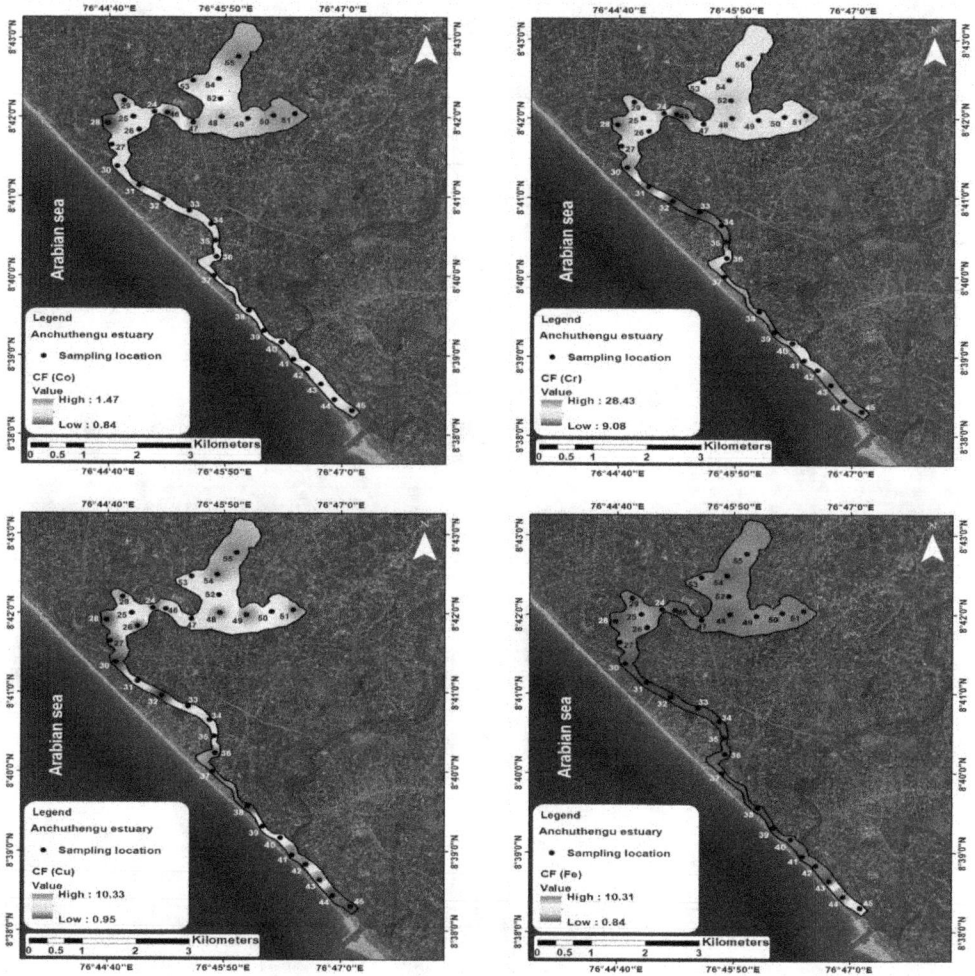

**Fig. 5.19** Spatial distribution map of the Contamination Factor (CF), in the surface sediments, Anchuthengu estuary, Kerala, India

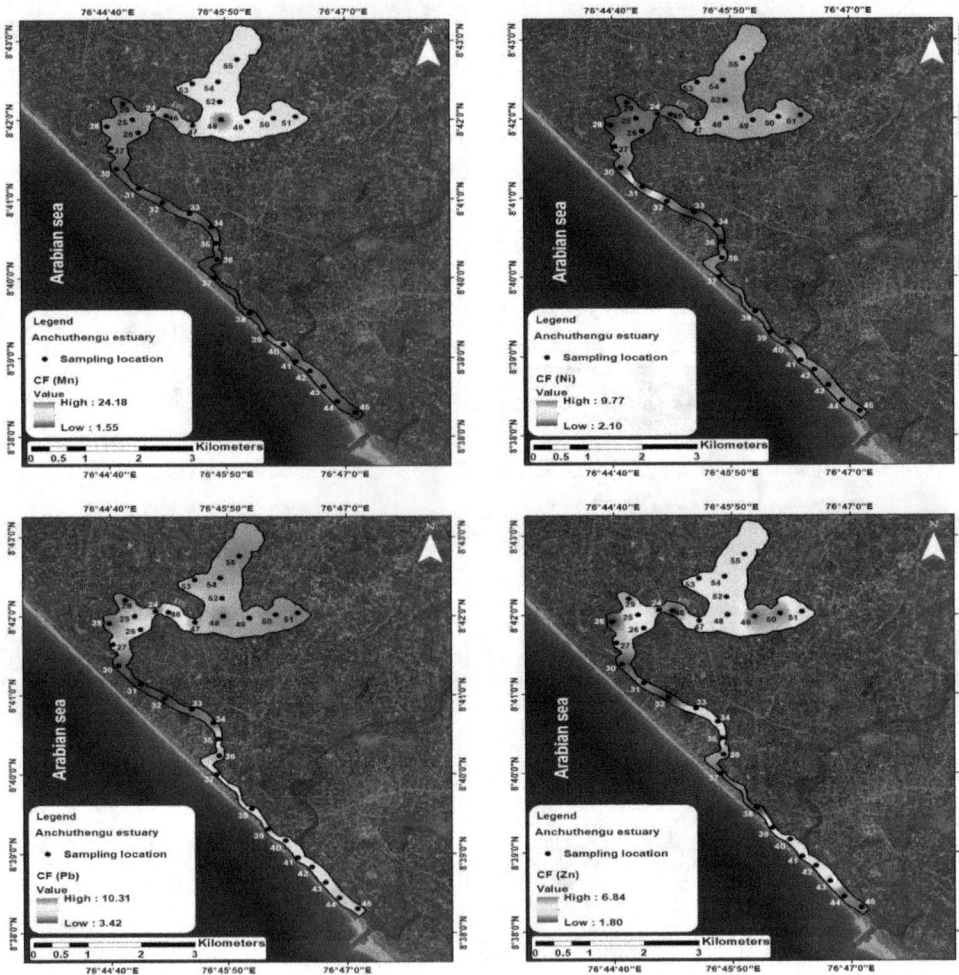

**Fig. 5.20** Spatial distribution map of the Contamination Factor (CF), in the surface sediments, Anchuthengu estuary, Kerala, India

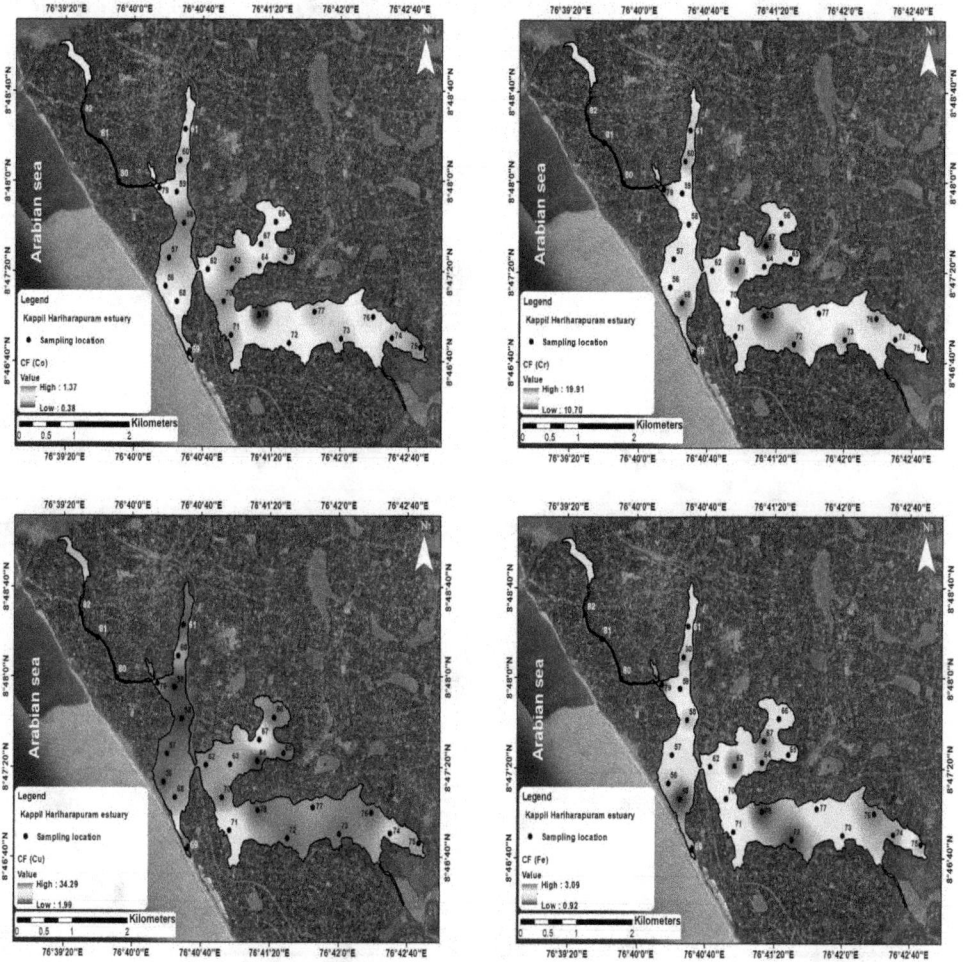

**Fig. 5.21** Spatial distribution map of the Contamination Factor (CF), in the surface sediments, Kappil - Hariharapuram estuary, Kerala, India

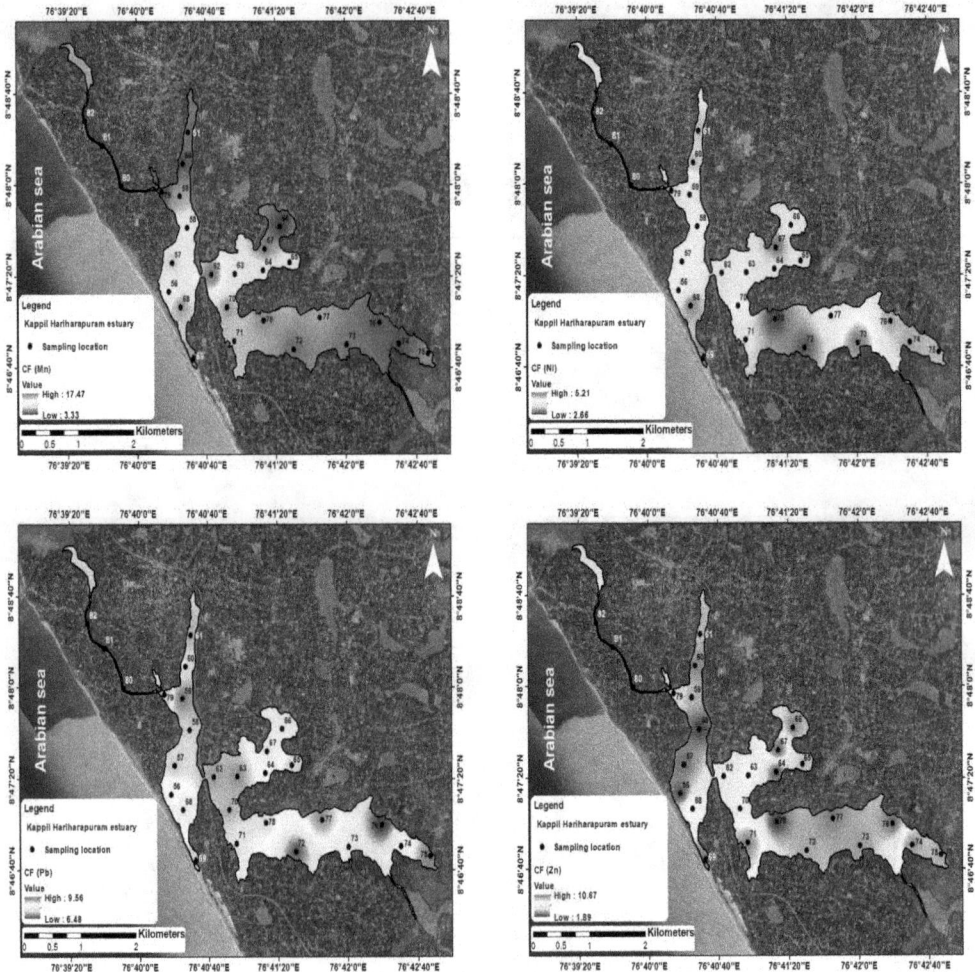

**Fig. 5.22** Spatial distribution map of the Contamination Factor (CF), in the surface sediments, Kappil - Hariharapuram estuary, Kerala, India

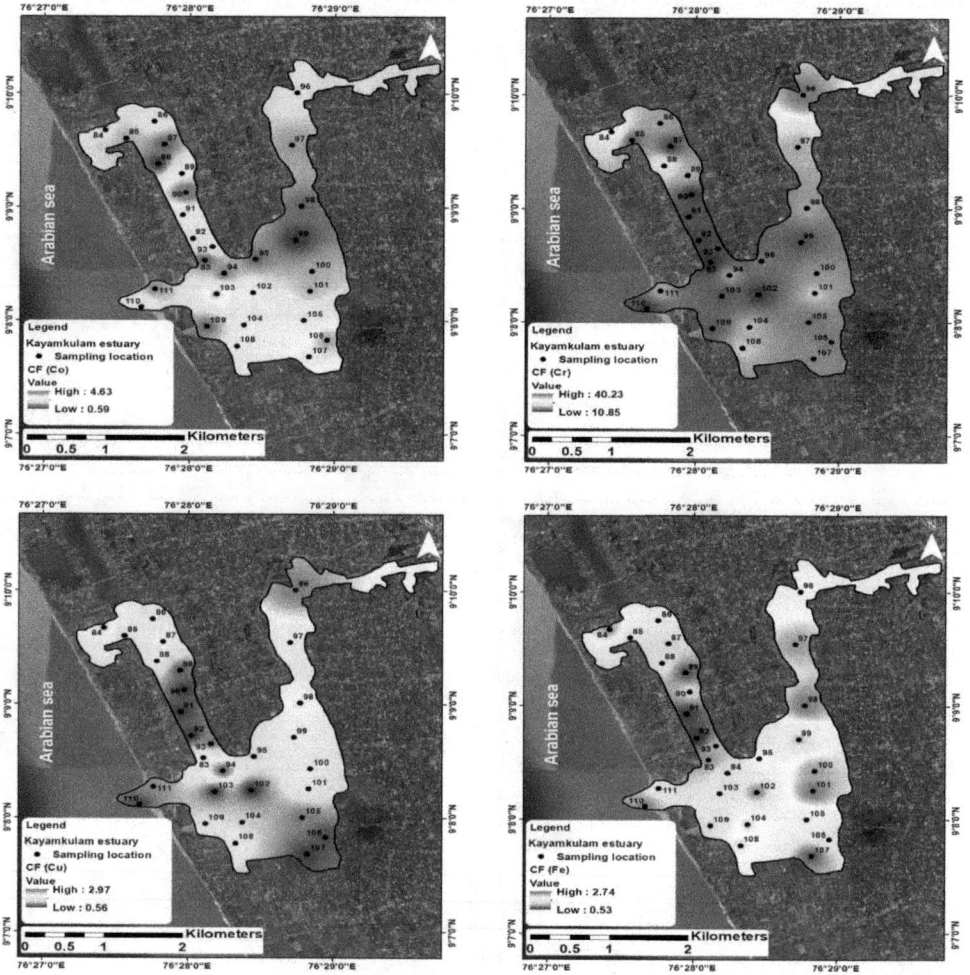

**Fig. 5.23** Spatial distribution map of the Contamination Factor (CF), in the surface sediments, Kayamkulam estuary, Kerala, India

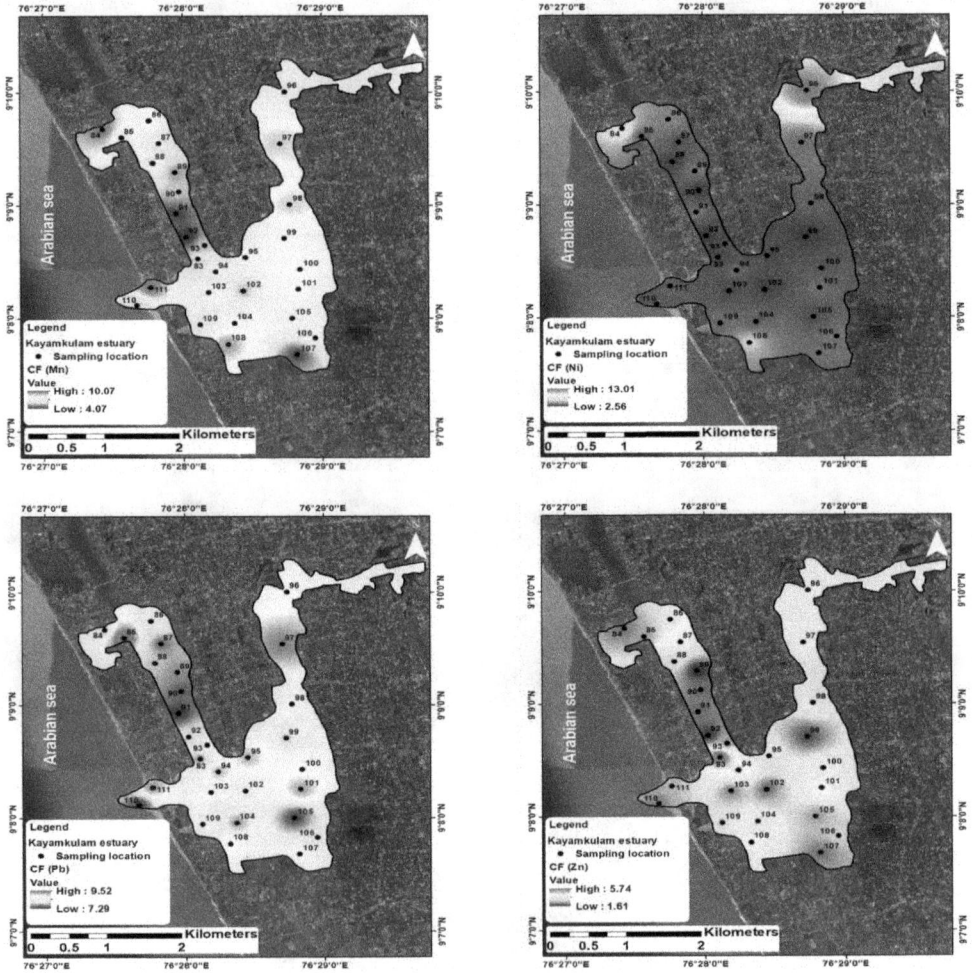

**Fig. 5.24** Spatial distribution map of the Contamination Factor (CF), in the surface sediments, Kayamkulam estuary, Kerala, India

Department of Geology, UNOM

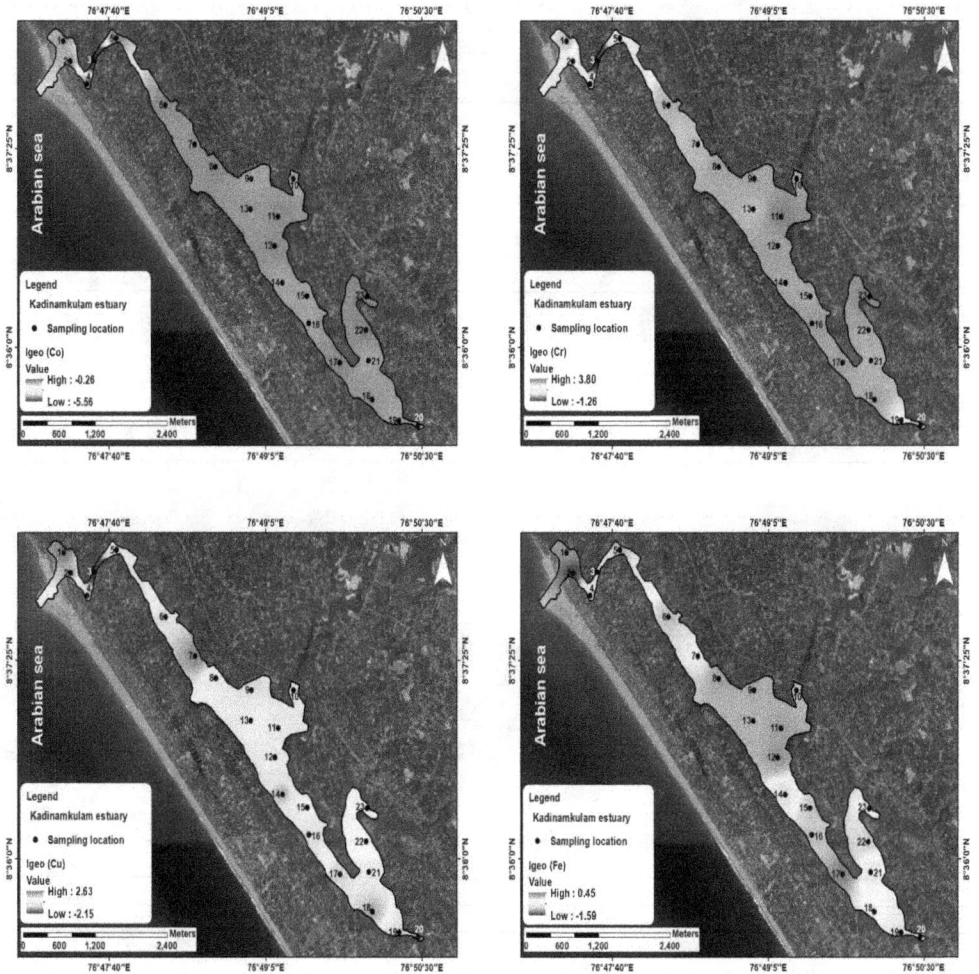

**Fig. 5.25** Spatial distribution map of the Geo-accumulation index (Igeo), in the surface sediments, Kadinamkulam estuary, Kerala, India

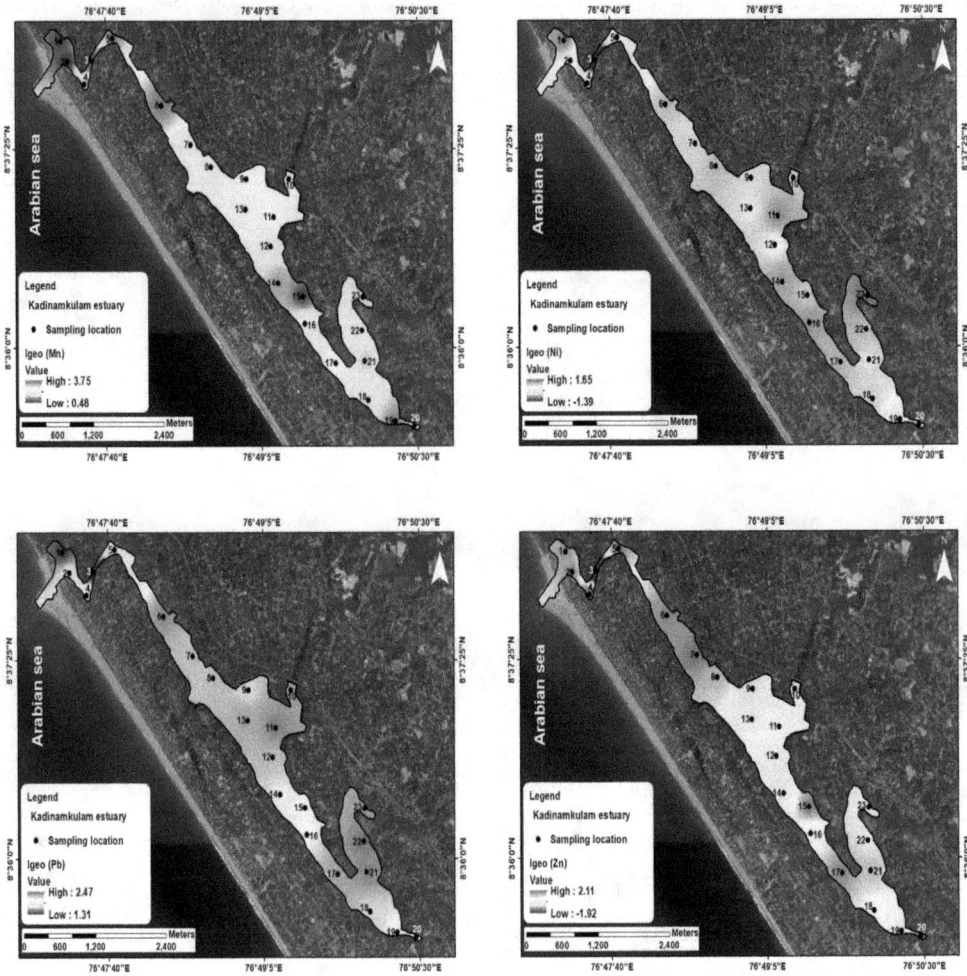

**Fig. 5.26** Spatial distribution map of the Geo-accumulation index (Igeo), in the surface sediments, Kadinamkulam estuary, Kerala, India

Department of Geology, UNOM

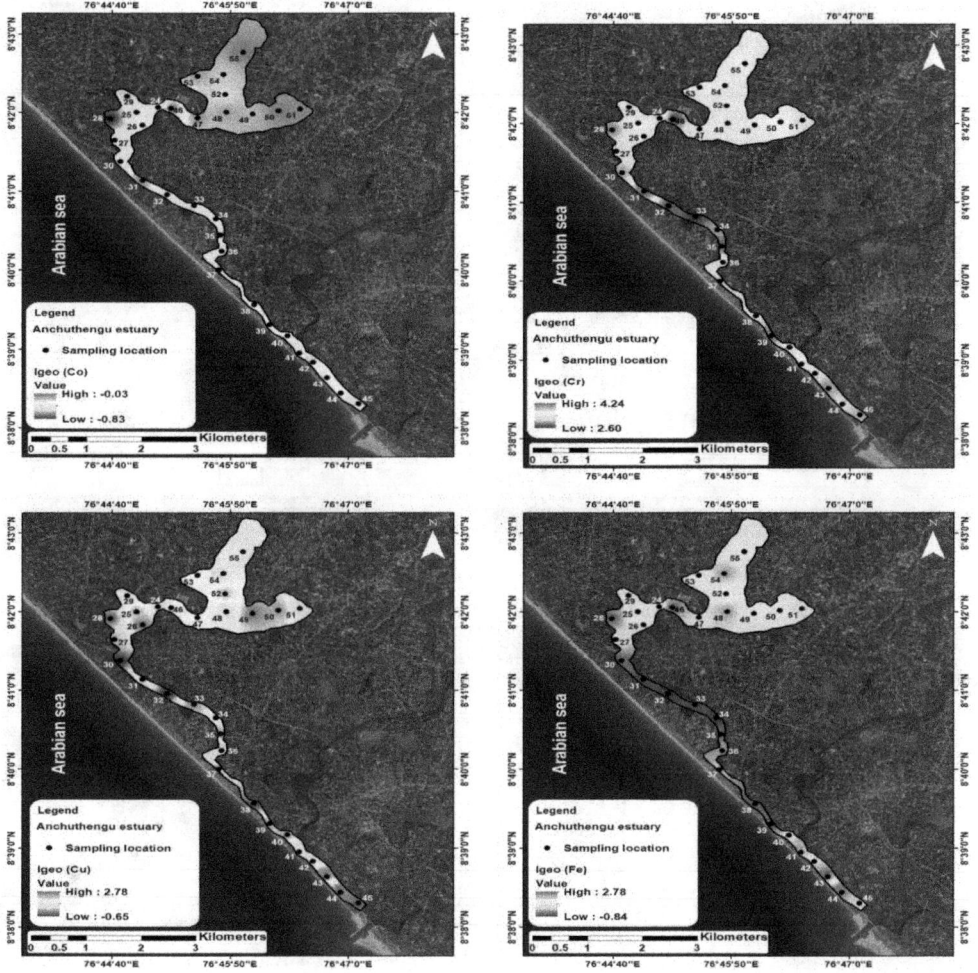

**Fig. 5.27** Spatial distribution map of the Geo-accumulation index (Igeo), in the surface sediments,
Anchuthengu estuary, Kerala, India

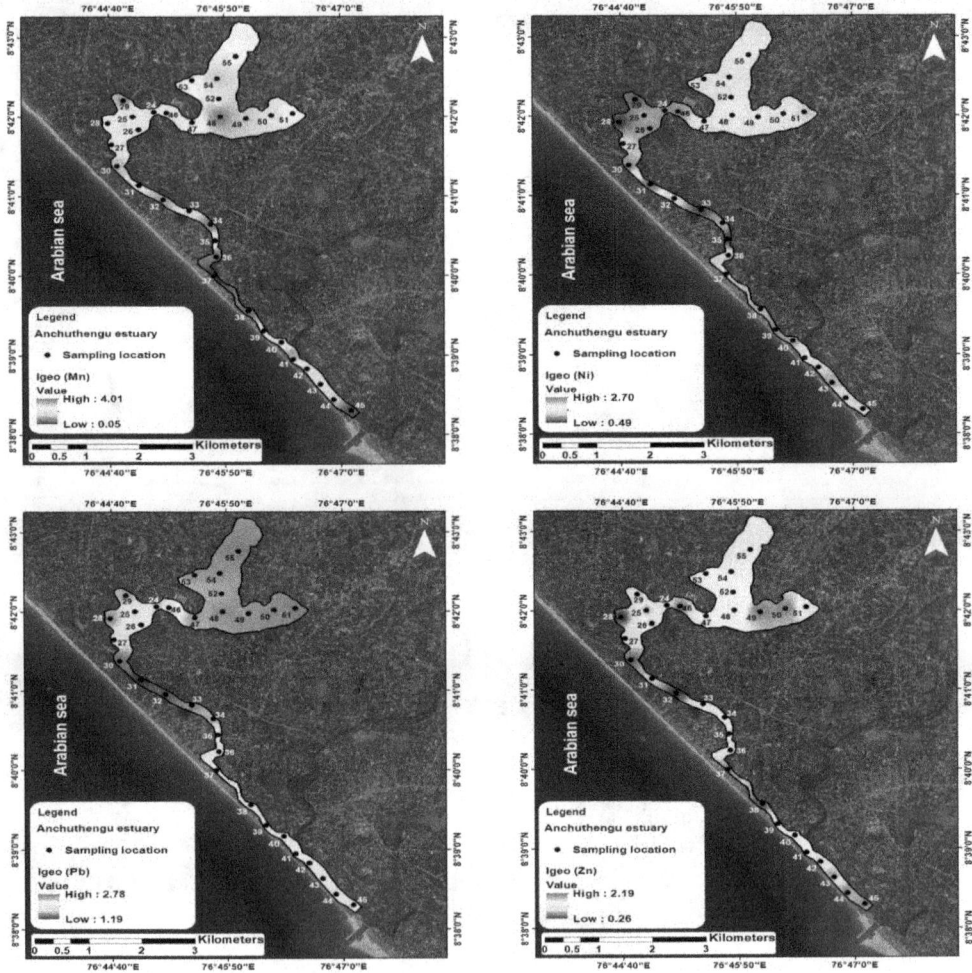

**Fig. 5.28** Spatial distribution map of the Geo-accumulation index (Igeo), in the surface sediments, Anchuthengu estuary, Kerala, India

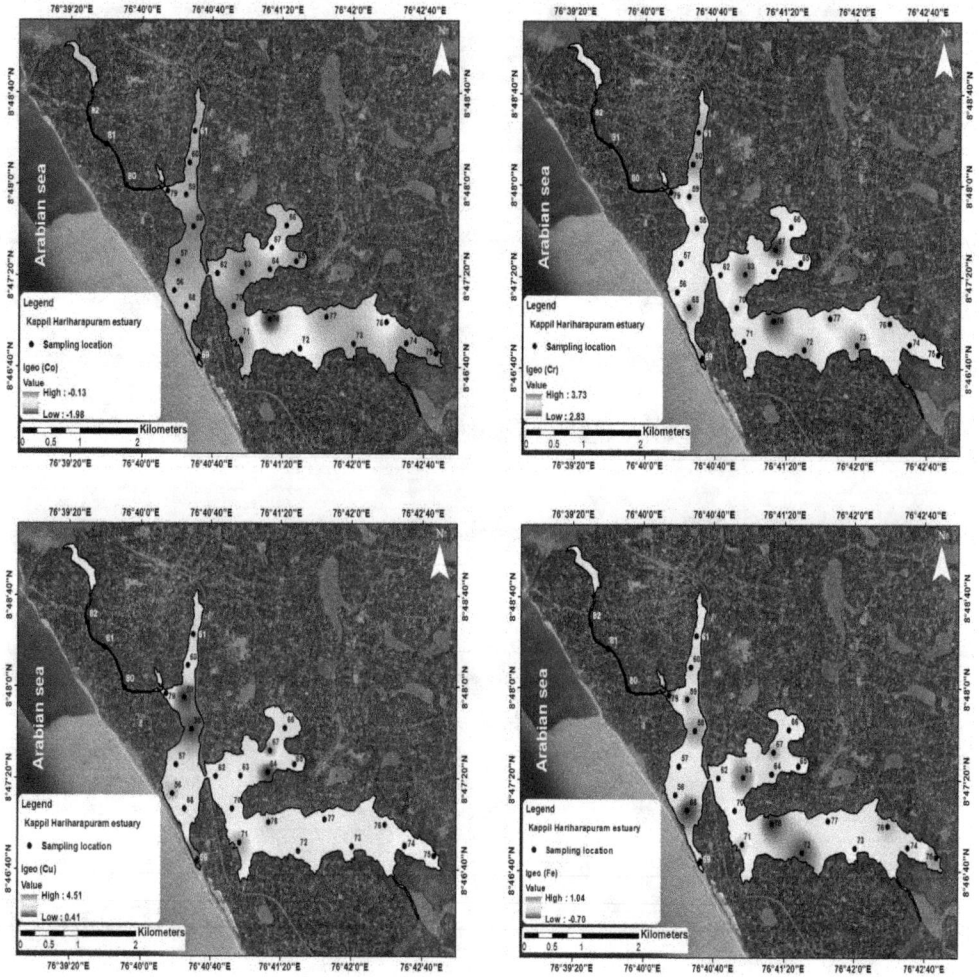

**Fig. 5.29** Spatial distribution map of the Geo-accumulation index (Igeo), in the surface sediments, Kappil – Hariharapuram estuary, Kerala, India

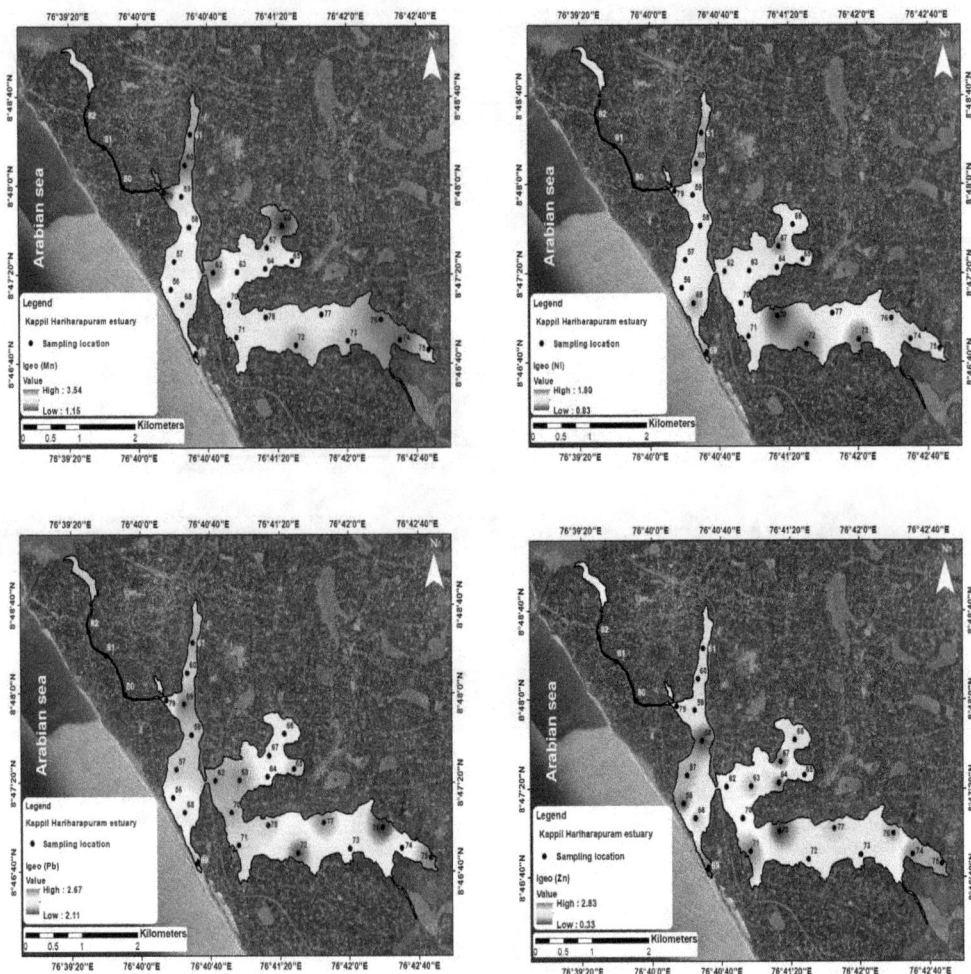

**Fig. 5.30** Spatial distribution map of the Geo-accumulation index (Igeo), in the surface sediments, Kappil – Hariharapuram estuary, Kerala, India

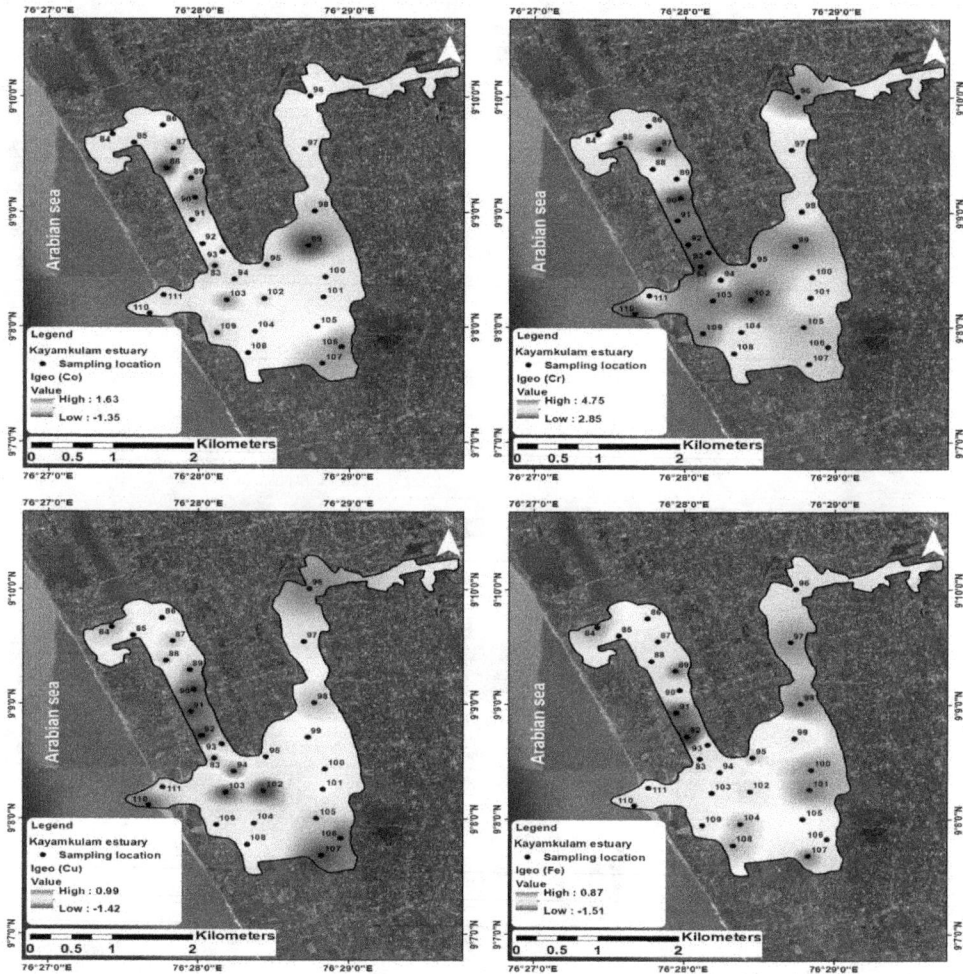

**Fig. 5.31** Spatial distribution map of the Geo-accumulation index (Igeo), in the surface sediments, Kayamkulam estuary, Kerala, India

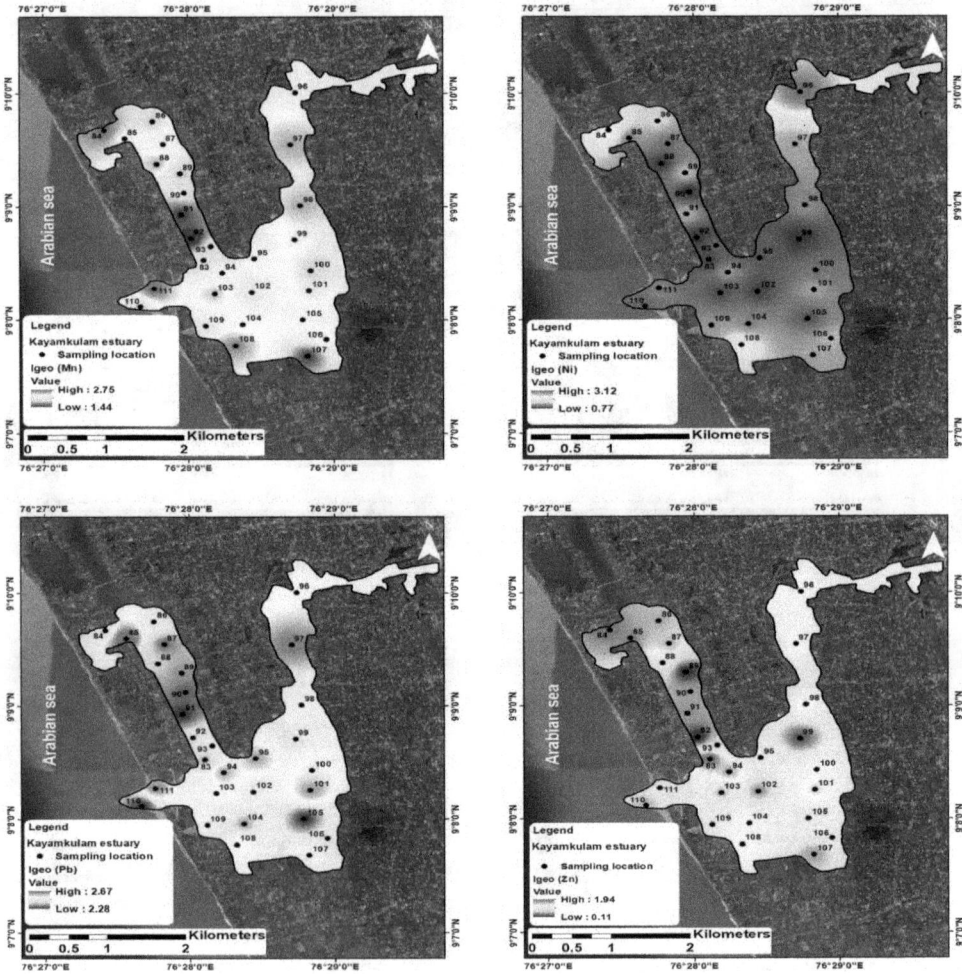

**Fig. 5.32** Spatial distribution map of the Geo-accumulation index (Igeo), in the surface sediments, Kayamkulam estuary, Kerala, India

Department of Geology, UNOM

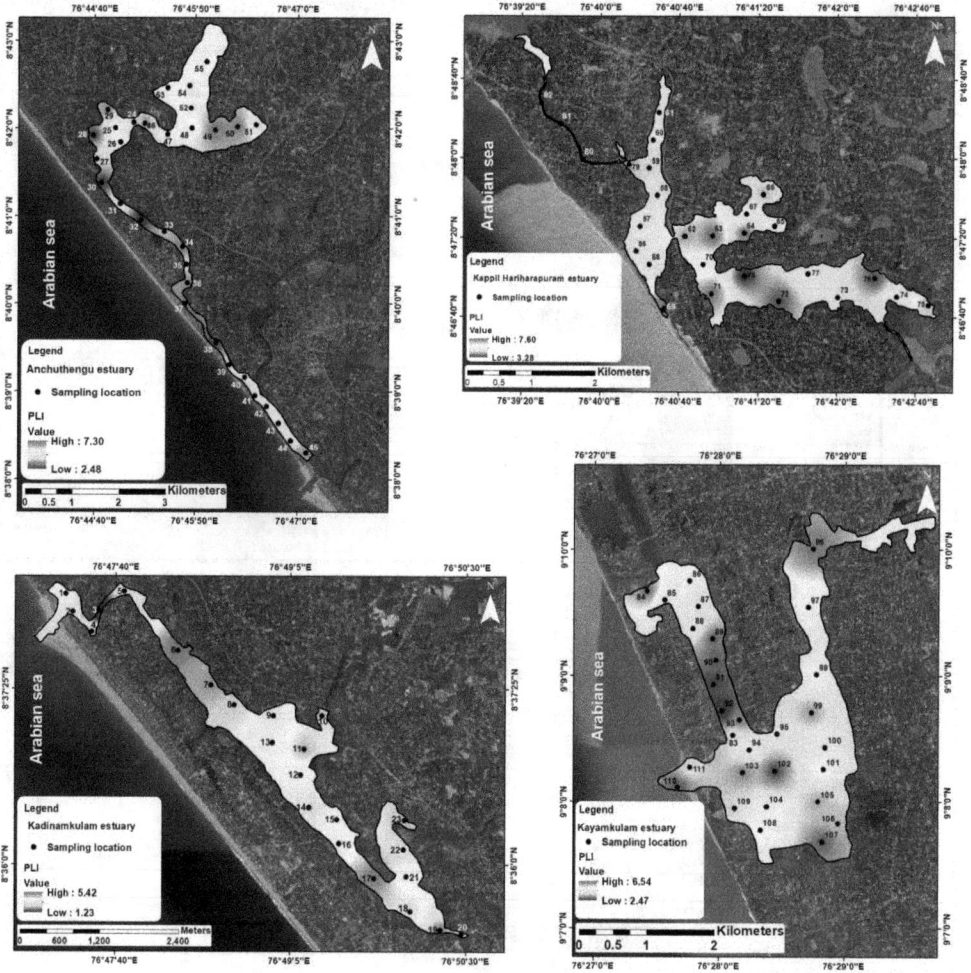

**Fig 5.33** Spatial distribution map of the Pollution Load Index (PLI), in the surface sediments of selected estuaries in Kerala, India

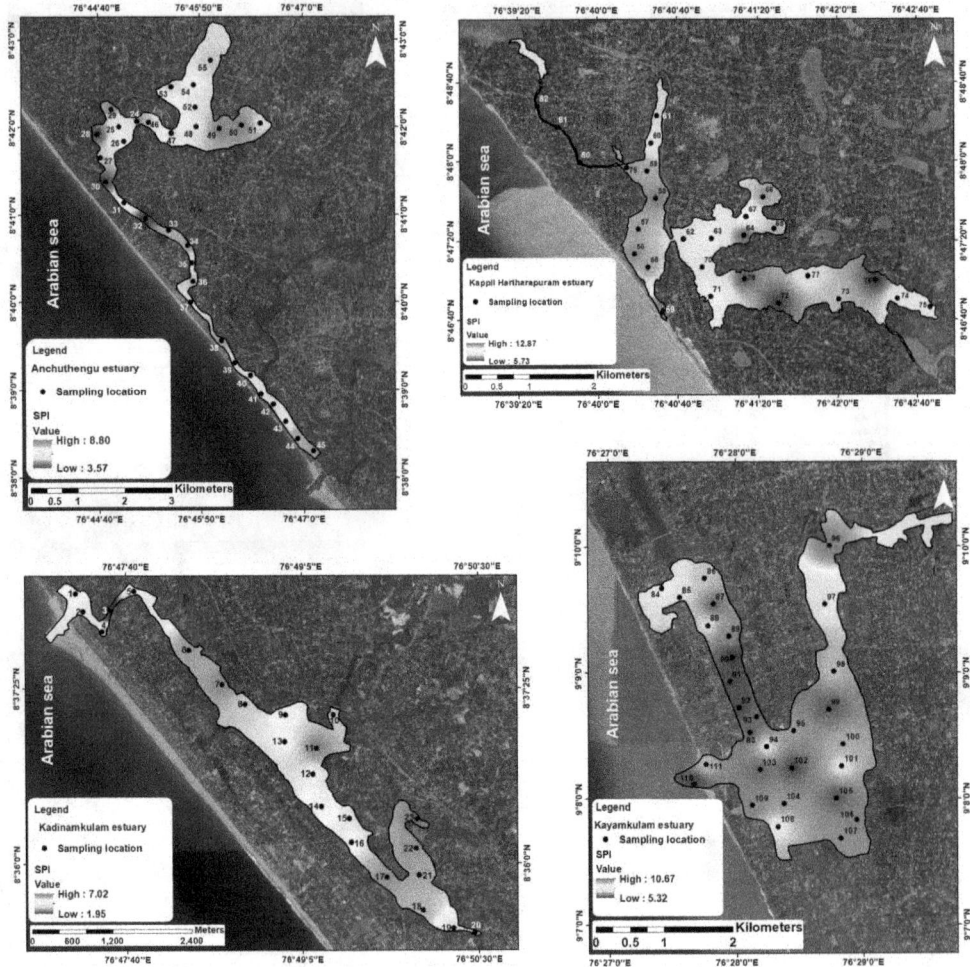

**Fig 5.34** Spatial distribution map of the Sediment Pollution Index (SPI), in the surface sediments of selected estuaries in Kerala, India

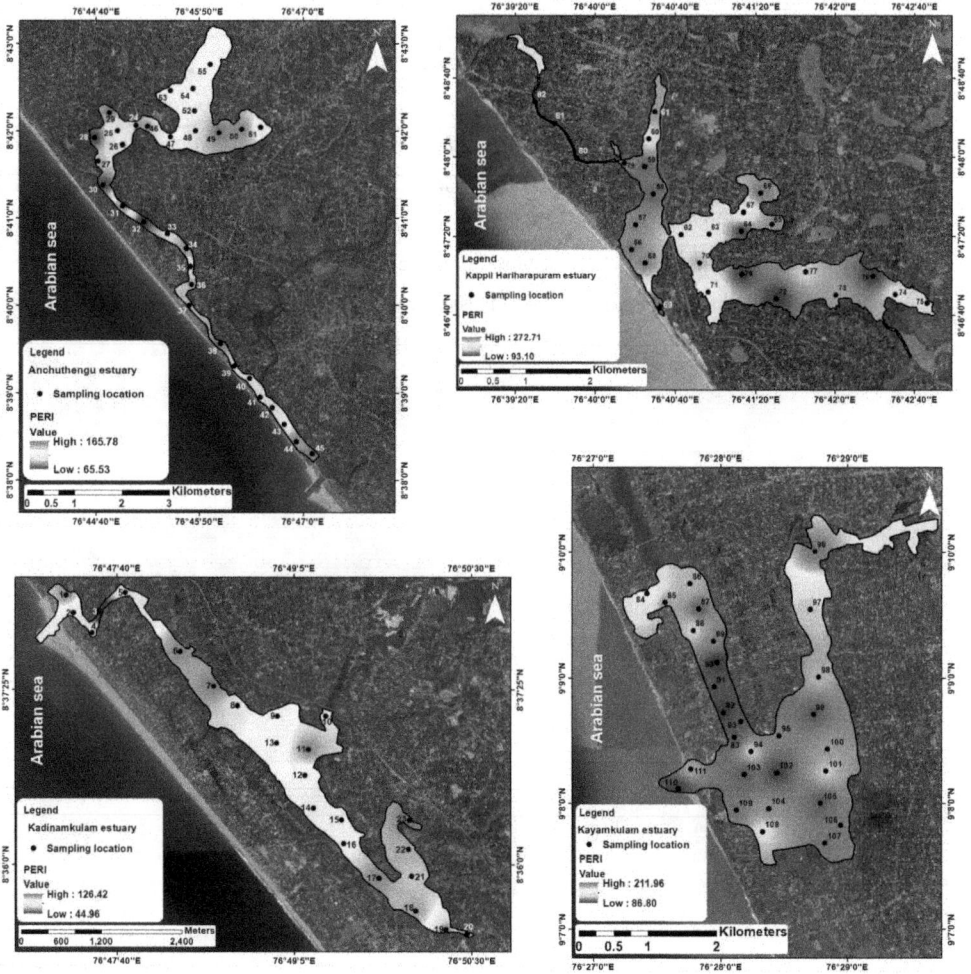

**Fig. 5.35** Spatial distribution map of the Potential Ecological Risk Index (PERI) in the surface sediments of selected estuaries in Kerala, India

## 5.4 COMPARISON OF TRACE ELEMENT CONCENTRATION WITH OTHER STUDIES IN ESTUARIES OF INDIA AND WORLD.

The trace element concentration in the estuarine surface sediments was compared with other estuaries in Indian and global scenario. The mean value for the present estuarine sediment's Fe and Mn value shows lower proportion whereas Ni, Pb, Zn, Cu, Co and Cr show higher proportion of the mean value for the present estuarine sediments when comparing to UCC and local background values. The trace element concentration of other estuaries compared shows varying values for metal to metal and also from location to location. Fe and Mn concentration of the present study with other compared studies shows majority of the compared studies has values higher than the present study. The concentration of the trace elements trend in the present study is noted to be lesser than Ashtamudi Lagoon (Hussain *et al.,* 2020), Vembanad Lake (Selvam *et al.,* 2012) and Estuaries of Nellore coast (Reddy *et al.,* 2016). (Table 5.13).

**Table. 5.13** Comparison table of average elements concentration from the present study, different coastal regions around the world and India

| S.No | Study Area | Fe | Mn | Pb | Zn | Cu | Cr | Ni | Co | References |
|------|-----------|-----|-----|-----|-----|-----|-----|-----|-----|-----------|
| 1 | Ashtamudi Lagoon, SW coast of India | 66387.9 | 1288.4 | 113.3 | 112.2 | 53.1 | 942.1 | 115 | 32.9 | **Hussain et al., 2020** |
| 2 | Vemabanad Lake, SW coast of India | 54000 | 440.7 | 35.3 | 208.8 | 31.5 | 110.7 | 48.2 | 19.3 | **Selvam et al., 2012** |
| 3 | Pulicat Lagoon, SE coast of India | 35572.9 | 247.8 | 30.4 | 96.5 | 29.6 | 206.9 | 98.8 | NA | **Saravanan et al., 2018** |
| 4 | Pitchavaram Estuary, SE coast of India | 32482 | 941 | 11.2 | 93 | 43.4 | 141.2 | 62 | 35.3 | **Ramanathan et al., 1999** |
| 5 | Punnakayal Estuary, SE coast of India | 28363 | 277.6 | 28.13 | 231 | 30.98 | 9.34 | 21.2 | 3.65 | **Magesh et al., 2018** |
| 6 | Estuaries of Nellore coast, Andhra Pradesh | 1498.5 | 13.84 | 159.6 | 234.7 | 197.8 | 55.42 | 71.63 | 4.98 | **Reddy et al., 2016** |
| 7 | Klang Estuary, Malaysia | NA | 105±16.17 | 37.39±17.22 | 22.46±18.8 | 9.38±10.73 | NA | NA | NA | **El Turk et al., 2019** |
| 8 | Can Gio mangrove estuary, Vietnam | 55302 | 1055 | 21 | NA | 33 | 79 | 38 | 13 | **Thanh-Nho et al., 2018** |
| 9 | Selected estuaries in South west coast of Kerala (Mean value) | 25084.86 | 283.01 | 84.57 | 138.34 | 76.66 | 284.95 | 123.63 | 42.60 | **Present study** |
| | Kadinamkulam | 19893.76 | 242.91 | 76.48 | 130.96 | 66.57 | 251.61 | 112.30 | 33.02 | |
| | Anchuthengu | 30842.49 | 279.61 | 73.55 | 122.58 | 71.23 | 272.58 | 119.73 | 39.04 | |
| | Kappil – Hariharapuram | 26037.23 | 292.69 | 95.91 | 192.07 | 143.74 | 283.84 | 127.36 | 35.17 | |
| | Kayamkulam | 23565.98 | 316.81 | 92.33 | 107.75 | 25.09 | 331.77 | 135.11 | 63.15 | |
| 10 | Background concentration | 36040.63 | 291.43 | 28.22 | 53.81 | 33.60 | 33.80 | 44.50 | 40.69 | **Jeshma 2020** (unpublished thesis) |
| 11 | UCC | 35000 | 600 | 20 | 71 | 25 | 35 | 20 | 10 | **Taylor and McLenan 1985** |

# CHAPTER-VI
# DISTRIBUTION OF MICROPLASTICS IN SEDIMENT SUBSTRATES

The plastic products are ideally suitable for a variety of applications for their low cost, excellent oxygen/moisture barrier properties, bio-inertness and light weight make them as an excellent packaging material. World annual production of plastics has increased by nearly 20-fold since the 1950s and reached 322 million metric tons in 2015 (Plastics Europe, 2015; Xiong *et al.,* 2018). The initial report of ocean plastic litter was reported during the 1970s and drew an attention of the scientific community (Carpenter *et al.,* 1972; Colton and Knapp, 1974; Coe and Rogers, 2012). Land-based sources, including beach litter contribute approximately 80% of the plastic debris. Among these, nearly 18% of the marine plastic debris found in the ocean environment is attributed to the fishing sector (Andrady, 2011). Aquaculture sector can also contribute the plastics to the marine environment and the rest of the things derived from land-based sources (Hinojosa and Thiel, 2009). According to the previously published researches, the size ranges from 0.5 mm to 5 mm were constituted as a macro or meso plastics (Andrady, 2011; Cole *et al.,* 2011). However, the term 'microplastics' and 'micro-litter' has been defined differently by various researchers. According to Gregory and Andrady (2003) micro-litter has been defined as the barely visible particles that pass through a 500 μm sieve, but retained by a 67 μm sieve (~0.06–0.5 mm in diameter), while particles range from few μm to 500 μm were called microplastics. Microplastics may cause potential risk to the aquatic environment due to their long residence time, possible to ingest by the biota and liberation of toxic components during degradation (Andrady, 2011; Rochman *et al.,* 2016; Axelsson *et al.,* 2017).

The relative systematic studies of marine and marginal marine environment associated microplastic were widely reported in India and around the world (Rochman and Hoellein, 2020; Vidyasakar *et al.,* 2018; Naidu *et al.,* 2018; Sruthy and Ramasamy, 2017; Syakti *et al.,* 2017; Tamminga *et al.,* 2018; Abayomi *et al.,* 2017; Stolte *et al.,* 2015). Most of the research studies on the impact of microplastics have focused on the marine species, including fish (Lusher *et al.,* 2013; Neves *et al.,* 2015; Bellas *et al.,* 2016), corals (Hall *et al.,* 2015; Hankins *et al.,* 2018; Reichert *et al.,* 2018) and benthic invertebrates (Naidu *et al.,* 2018), fur seals (Eriksson and

Burton, 2003), ingestion of plastics by birds (Mallory, 2008; Cadee, 2002) and turtles (Mascarenhas *et al.*, 2004; Tomas *et al.*, 2002). The previous studies reported the distribution of microplastics in a beach environment (Robin *et al.*, 2020), benthos (Naidu *et al.*, 2018) and surface sediments of estuaries (Sruthy and Ramasamy 2017), from the middle part of the Kerala, India. However, no comprehensive studies have been carried out in the estuarine sediments of southern Kerala. The aim of the present study is to assess the surface sediment associated microplastics from selected estuaries of Southern Kerala, India.

## 6.1 POTENTIAL SOURCES OF MICROPLASTICS (MPs)

Both land-based and sea-based sources of microplastics have been found in sediments throughout the Indian coast (Veerasingam *et al.*, 2016). The polymer varieties and abundance of MPs along the Indian coast demonstrate a strong correlation with inland sources like industrialization and urbanisation, as well as marine sources like fishing and shipping. In 2016, India's Central Pollution Control Board estimated that 62 metric tonnes of solid waste were produced, with 82 percent being collected (processed and discarded) and 18 percent being treated as litter (CPCB, 2016). If urban local bodies proceed to depend on landfill route for the Municipal Solid Waste management, by 2051 generation of the solid wastes will reach around 300 million tons annually (Joshi and Ahmed, 2016). Leachate mismanagement and uncontrolled flows of materials caused by open dumping results in surface water pollution. The major potential source of MPs could be the densely populated and urbanized coastal regions around the Indian Ocean (Li *et al.*, 2021).

Microplastics abundance and their composition along the Indian coast show higher diversity in river mouths and metropolitan cities, proving localized human activities influencing the MPs pollution in the nearshore marine environment. Veerasingam *et al.* (2017) states that almost 20% of the plastic debris are sea-based sources entering into the Indian Ocean. MP along the Indian coast were plastic debris originated from fisheries and aquaculture. Potential fishing areas in the Indian coast were noted with adverse effects of plastic debris in recent days (Kaladharan *et al.*, 2020).

Forty-four samples (Kayamkulam – 17 out of 29 samples, Kappil and Hariharapuram – 9 out of 27 samples; Anchuthengu- 10 out of 32 samples; Kadinamkulam- 8 out of 23 samples) were selected for the microplastics study from the collected 111 estuarine sediments from the selected estuaries in Kerala (Fig. 6.1). The surface sediment samples were homogenized and carefully packed in glass bottles with metal lid to avoid the contamination. The wet samples were sieved through 5 mm mesh in order to remove large debris, and to retain particles of <5 mm size. The sediment was transferred to ceramic bowls and kept in the hot oven at 60˚C. The oven dried samples were homogenized and pass through the 5 mm testing sieve to remove the coarse debris and organic plant remains (Sruthy and Ramasamy, 2017). Extraction procedure for MPs from sieved sediment samples was done as per National Oceanic and Atmospheric Administration (NOAA) protocol (Masura *et al.*, 2015).

Accordingly, 30g of dried sediment was treated with 30% Hydrogen peroxide ($H_2O_2$) solution followed by 2N HCl to remove the organic matter and calcareous phase from the surface sediments. Later, density separation method was adopted as follows: The pre-treated estuarine sediments were thoroughly mixed with 50 ml of pre-prepared zinc chloride solution (density: 1.58 g/cm3). The mixture was filtered using 0.45 μm Whatman® nitrocellulose membrane filter paper and vacuum pump assembly. The filtration procedure was repeated three times for better extraction results. The filter paper was examined under optical stereo zoom microscope for microplastic distribution. The shape of the retained particles above filter paper was classified (Free *et al.*, 2014) as a fibre (thin or fibrous, straight plastic particles), pellet/beads (hard, rounded plastic particles), fragment (hard, jagged plastic particles), and film (thin plane of flimsy plastic particles).

To determine the separated polymer compositions, the Bruker Fourier-transform infrared spectroscopy (FTIR) method was used in conjunction with an Attenuated Total Reflectance (ATR) diamond crystal attachment to investigate the composition of the microplastics. The microplastic compositions frequency curve was identified using a readily available spectral library with instrument setup. The extracted microplastic was classified based on the colour, shape and composition of the materials under the optical stereo zoom microscope-Polarizing mode with online digital camera setup (Model – NIKON SMZ25). The microplastic distribution in terms of colour, shape, size and composition were represented in the pie chart. The graphical representations were prepared using Microsoft Excel software package (Microsoft office, 2007).

The blank measurement procedure was performed to reduce the error percentage during sample processing and microscopic examination of microplastic pollution (Dris *et al.*, 2016). The cotton lab coats and surgical rubber clauses were used throughout the study. All the analytical processes were performed in a stainless-steel laminar flow bench and the laminar flow bench was periodically clean with alcoholic wipes. All glassware's were thoroughly rinsed with double distilled water in order to avoid contamination with airborne MPs. The replicate (2 times) study was conducted during microplastic extraction and identification to minimize the error percentage. Simultaneously, the blank measurement was carried out to eliminate the external/airborne microplastic contribution during the investigation. The blank measurement shows negative results, and the absence of microplastic contamination in the lab environment.

This study found totally 628 microplastic particles in the surface sediments of the selected estuaries. Among these, 117 MPs found from the Kadinamkulam estuary, 182 MPs found from the Anchuthengu estuary, 108 MPs found from the Kappil- Hariharapuram estuary and 221 MPs found from the Kayamkulam estuary falling under three different microplastic shapes (Fibres, Films and Fragments). The highest microplastic distribution was found at station 103 at the mouth of the Kayamkulam estuary. The mouth of the estuary has sandy sediment substrate, whereas the other stations were dominated by clay and sandy silt sediments, and the interstices present in the sand grains allow the microplastics to accommodate themselves in the sediments (Govender *et al.*, 2020). Salinity-induced gravitational circulation was the main cause of sedimentation in this estuary (Srinivas *et al.*, 2010), thus being the major source of circulation of microplastics in the estuary than flowing water. Hence, the flowing water in the estuary has a low flow rate

## 6.2 COLOR OF MPs

The colour classification of the microplastic was classified under two broad groups such as white and coloured plastic. The MP with various colors in the sediment is originated from the use of colored plastic products in the daily life, such as clothing, packaging, fishing (Zhang *et al.*, 2015). However, the colors can change due to weathering (Wu *et al.*, 2018) during transport in the surface water. In Kadinamkulam estuary, the white and coloured microplastics occupy 19.66% and 80.34%, respectively. White microplastics occupy 22% and coloured microplastics occupy 78% in the total microplastic distribution in Anchuthengu and Kappil- Hariharapuram estuaries. In Kayamkulam estuary, white and colour plastic occupied nearly 44.34% and 55.66% in the total microplastic count, respectively (Table. 6.1- 6.4; Fig. 6.1 & 6.2). The colour varieties were dominated in the total count of microplastic except few locations (S.no 98, 99 and 101).

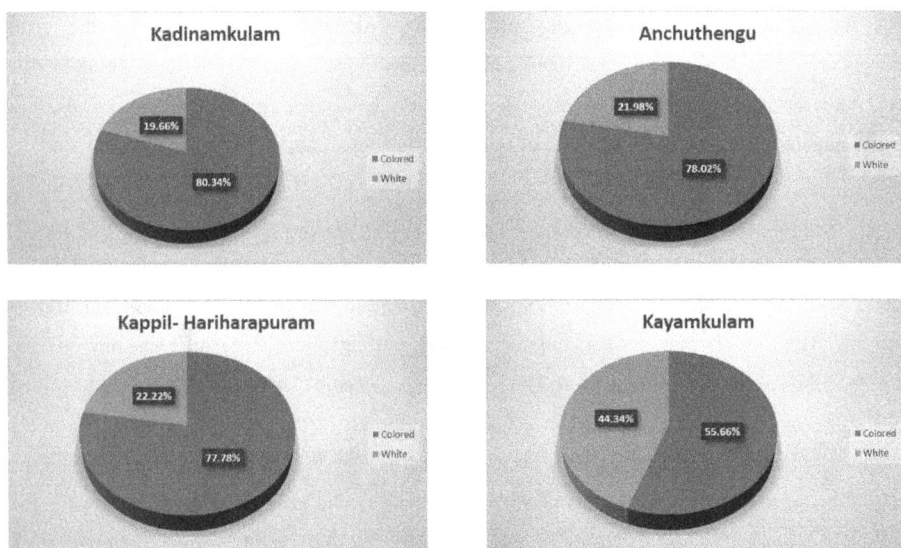

**Fig. 6.1** Chart representing the colour classification of microplastic in the surface sediments of the selected estuaries in Kerala

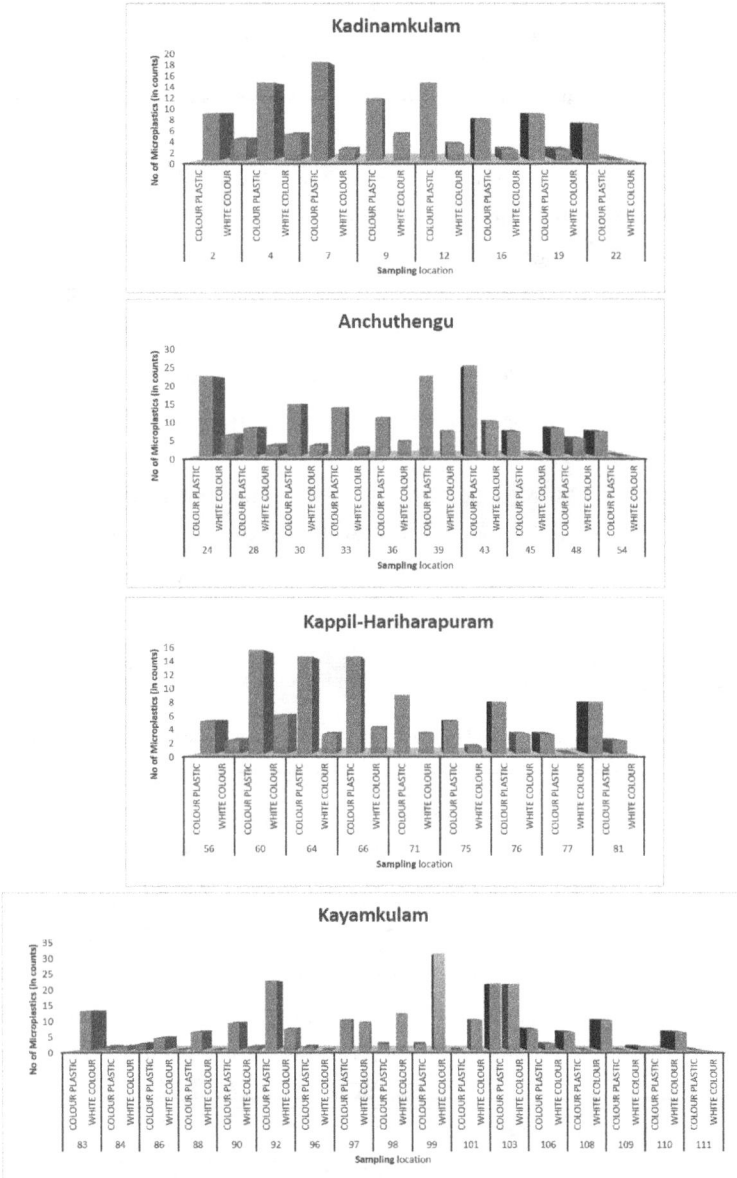

**Fig. 6.2** Chart representing the colour classification of microplastic in the surface sediments

## 6.3 SIZE OF MPs

Local climatic variables, such as thermal decomposition, transit, distance from the source, and time spent in the aquatic/marine environment, are primarily responsible for microplastic size (Zhao *et al.*, 2015; Naidu *et al.*, 2018). The size and distribution of the MPs were controlled by the durability of the plastics, physical factors (wave action, winds, etc.) and intensity of the UV light (Thompson *et al.*, 2004; Barnes *et al.*, 2009). The size classification of the of microplastic suggests that the majority of the particles falling under < 1000 μm (68.94%) followed by 1000 to 2000 μm (21.97%). The similar observation was observed in the Kayamkulam (<1000 μm −62.89%; 1000 to 2000 μm − 29.86% and >3000 μm − 7.23%) and the Kappil- Hariharapuram estuary (<1000 μm −70.37%; 1000 to 2000 μm − 21.30%); slightly higher in the Anchuthengu estuary (<1000 μm − 72.53%; 1000 to 2000 μm − 16.48%) and Kadinamkulam estuary (< 1000 μm (74.35%) followed by 1000 to 2000 μm (16.23%); (Table. 6.1- 6.4; Fig. 6.3 & 6.4). Microplastics may enter and be transferred along marine food webs through planktivorous fish species, because small planktonic organisms are particularly susceptible to accidental ingestion of microplastics suspended in the water column (Moore *et al.*, 2002).

## 6.4 SHAPE OF MPs

According to Doyle *et al.* (2011) and Hidalgo-Ruz *et al.* (2012), plastics were classified into four main groups: Fibres, Films, Fragments, and Pellets. In all the four estuaries' fibres were the dominant microplastic shape followed by fragment and filament. The fibre shape of the microplastic was dominated in the sediments (50.61%) followed by fragment shaped (40.29%) in the total distribution (Table. 6.1- 6.4; Fig. 6.5 & 6.6). The high-density plastic varieties like polypropylene and polyethylene were occupied maximum percentage in fragment and film shape particles and they dominated, where the sampling point is close to the households and transportation route (S.no 9, 12, 24, 39, 43, 48, 56, 75, 81, 90, 92, 98 & 101). Naidu *et al.* (2018) stated that the high-density polymer sinks and accumulate in the sediment. The distribution of these microplastics is primarily controlled by hydrographic factors such as surface currents, wave movements, and winds.

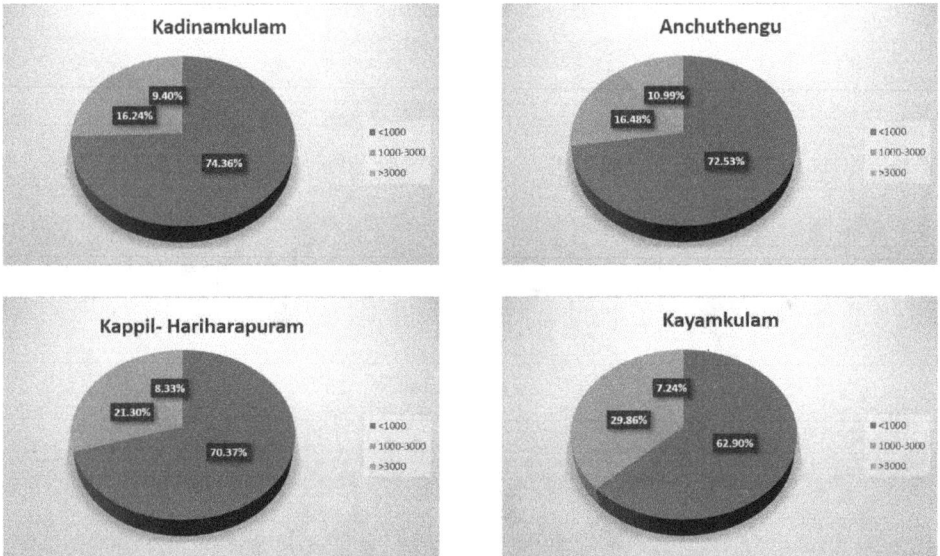

**Fig. 6.3** Chart representing the size classification of microplastic in the surface sediments of the selected estuaries in Kerala (in μm)

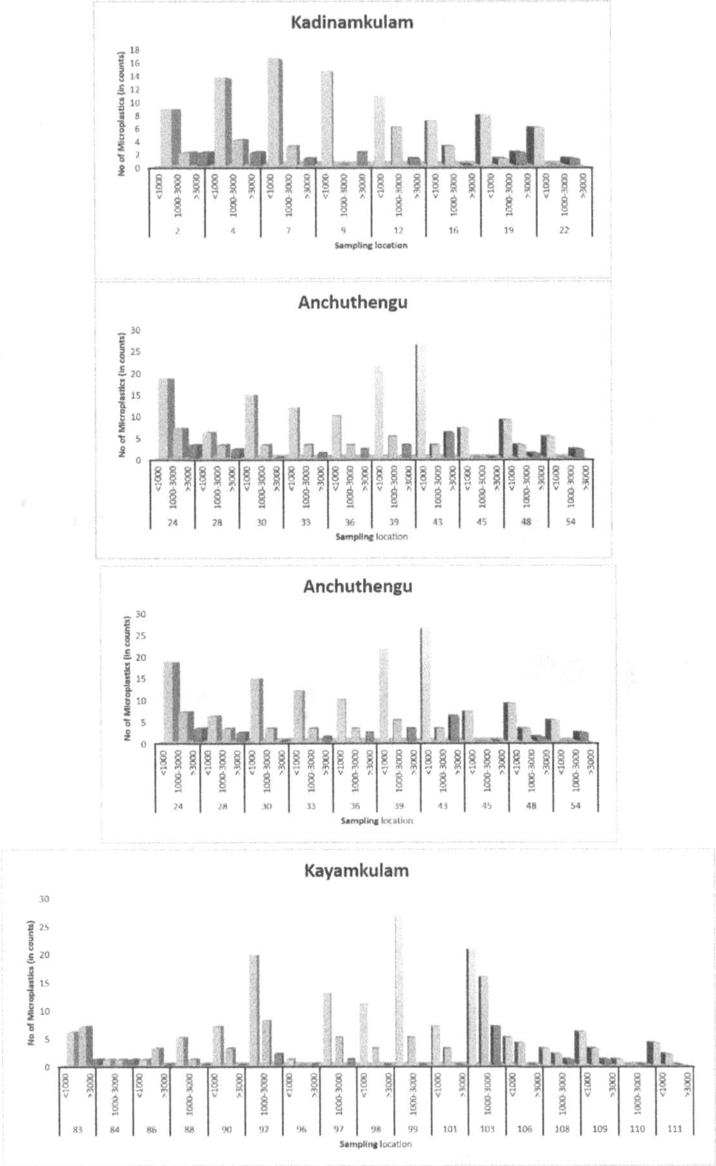

**Fig. 6.4** Chart representing the Size classification of microplastic in the surface sediments, (in μm)

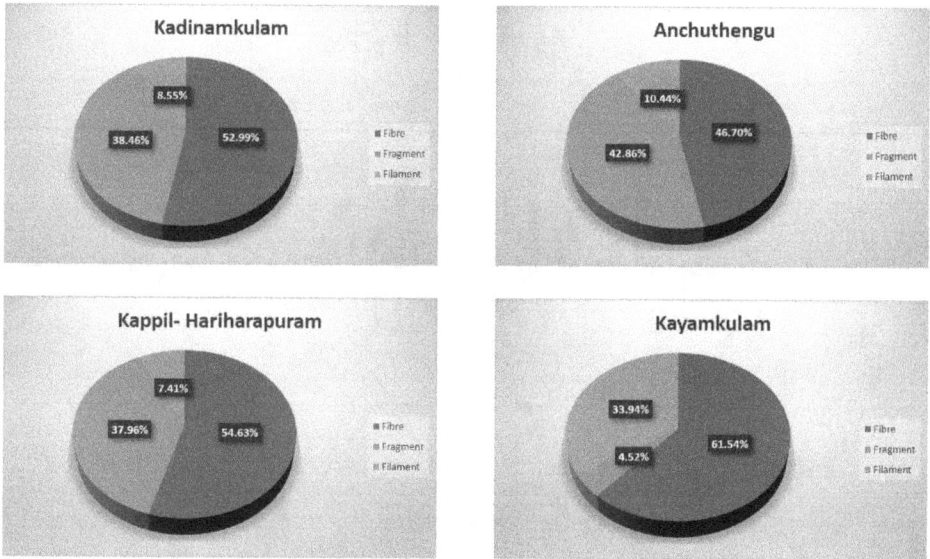

**Fig. 6.5** Chart representing the shape classification of microplastic in the surface sediments of the selected estuaries in Kerala

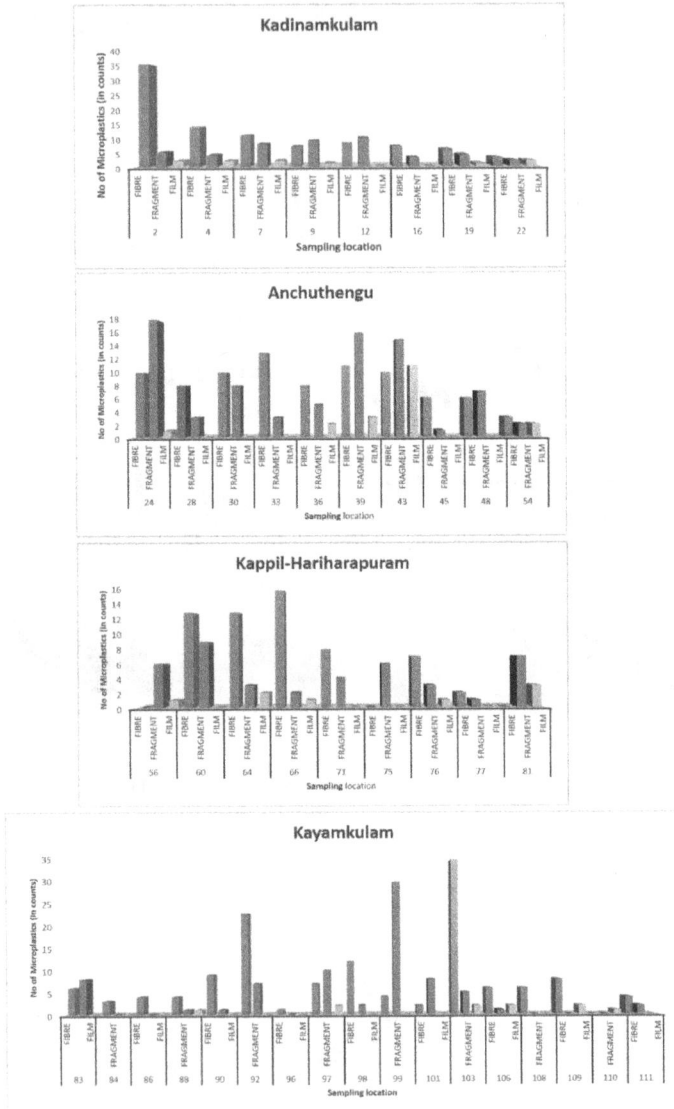

**Fig. 6.6** Chart representing the shape classification of microplastic in the surface sediments of the selected estuaries in Kerala

## 6.5 CHARACTERIZATION OF MPs

The chief sources of MPs in marine ecosystems are rivers, maritime traffic, and fishing activities (Thiel *et al.*, 2013; Desforges *et al.*, 2014). According to Veerasingam *et al.* (2016), the extreme rainfall induced flood carry the terrestrial plastics to marine ecosystems through rivers. The microplastic compositions frequency curve was identified using a readily available spectral library with instrument setup. The polyester fibre (49.88%) found the highest prevalence among the other three polymer types (polyester-PY; polypropylene-PP; and polyethylene-PE). PE and PP also significantly contributed to the total distribution of the microplastics in the study area. The maximum distribution of PE and PP was found at stations 5, 9 and 14, respectively (Table. 6.1- 6.4; Fig. 6.7 & 6.8). When comparing Kayamkulam estuary to Kadinamkulam, Anchuthengu and Kappil- Hariharapuram estuaries, distribution of PE and PP were relatively higher in Kayamkulam than other three estuaries.

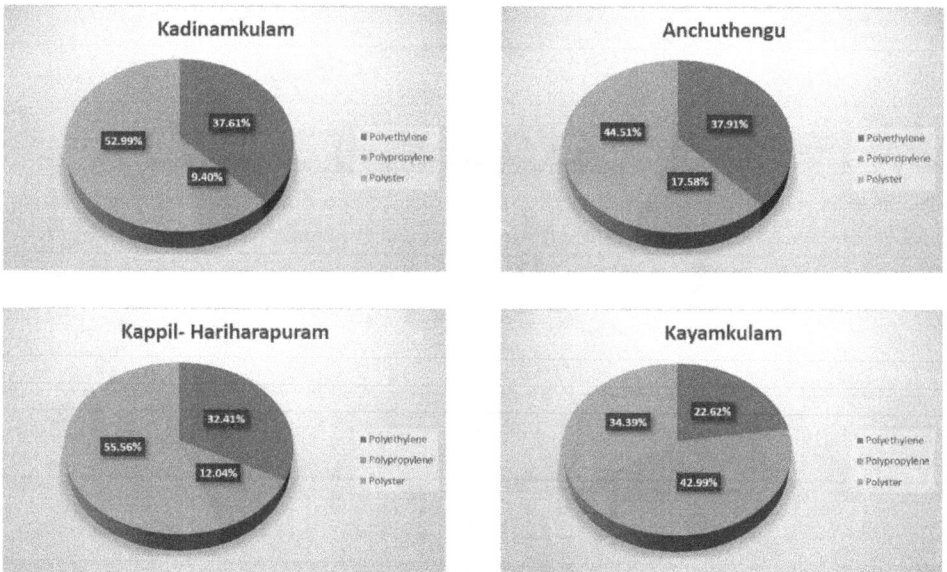

**Fig. 6.7** Chart representing the composition classification of microplastic in the surface sediments of the selected estuaries in Kerala

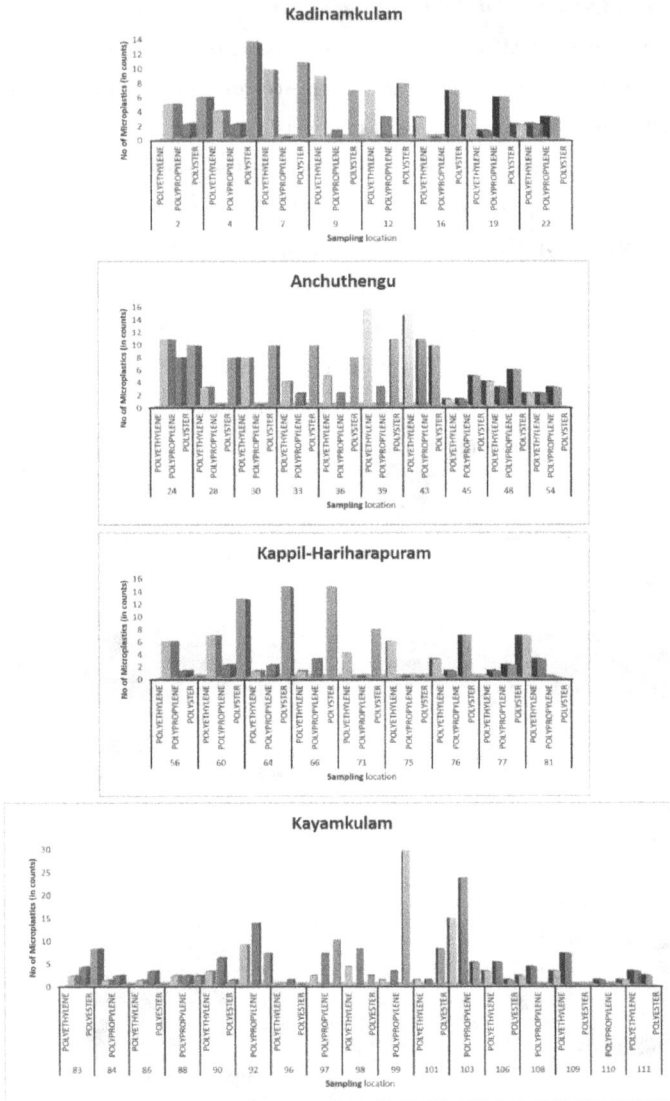

**Fig. 6.8** Chart representing the composition classification of microplastic in the surface sediments of the selected estuaries in Kerala

The overall distribution of microplastics in the surface sediments of selected estuaries in Kerala shown in Fig. 6.9. The overall microplastics were dominated by coloured plastic (79.01%) followed by white colour (20.99%). The size and shape classification suggest that they are conquered by < 1000 μm and fibre shape microplastic, respectively. The estuarine sediments were dominated by polyester (49.88), polyethylene (36.36%) followed by polypropylene (13.76%) (Fig 6.10).

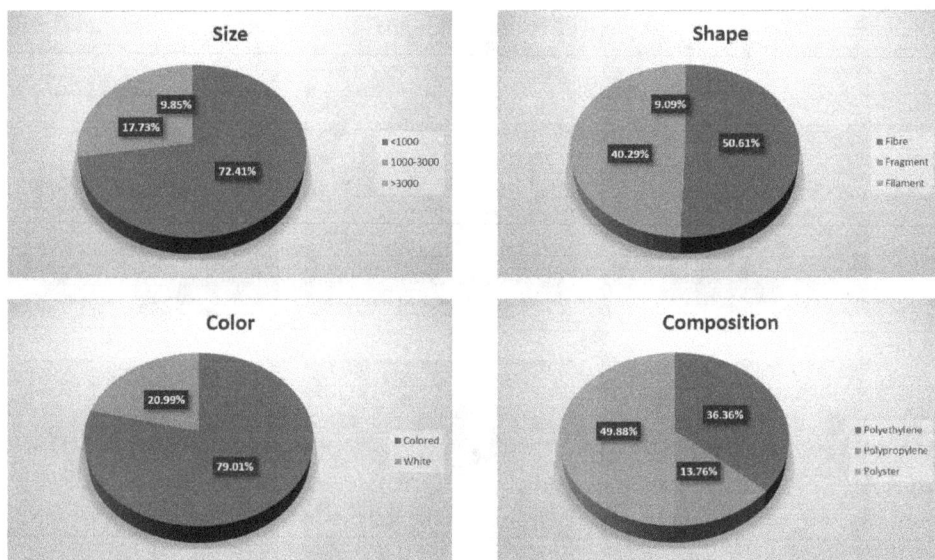

**Fig 6.9** Overall distribution of microplastics based on colour, shape, size, and composition (in %), from selected estuaries of Kerala

## 6.6 MICROMORPHOLOGY

Micromorphology features are useful in determining the impact of microplastic transport and breakdown. Photo, thermal, or biological degradation processes are the most common causes of polymer disintegration (Shah *et al.*, 2008; Retama *et al.*, 2016). The thickness and length of the microplastic fibres range from 4.517 to 21.247 μm and 0.36 to 10446 μm, respectively (Fig. 6.10). Due to prolonged exposure to sunlight and warmth, microplastic fibres originating from land-based activities disintegrated quickly (Cooper and Corcoran, 2010). In total, 13 microplastic particles were carefully chosen for FTIR analysis. The frequency curve of the microplastic compositions matched a readily available instrument spectral library by about 92.43 to 97.5 percent (Fig. 6.11). The photographs of microplastics form the selected estuaries captured under stereo-zoom binocular microscope were given (Fig 6.12 & 6.13)

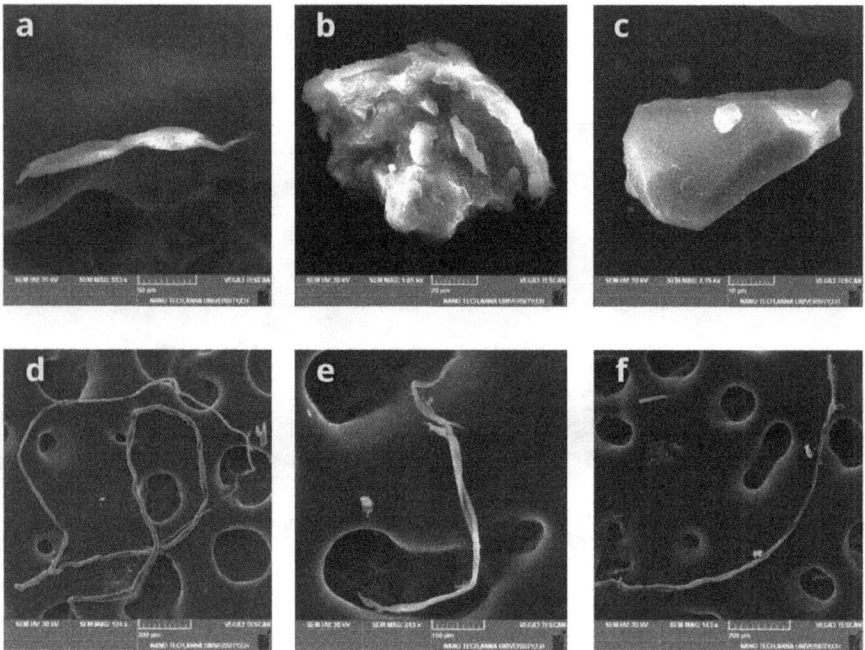

**Fig. 6. 10.** Showing film, fragment and fiber shape microplastic debris (**a.** Film – polyethylene; **b & c** – Fragment, polypropylene; **d, e & f.** Fiber – polystyrene with fine embedded impurities)

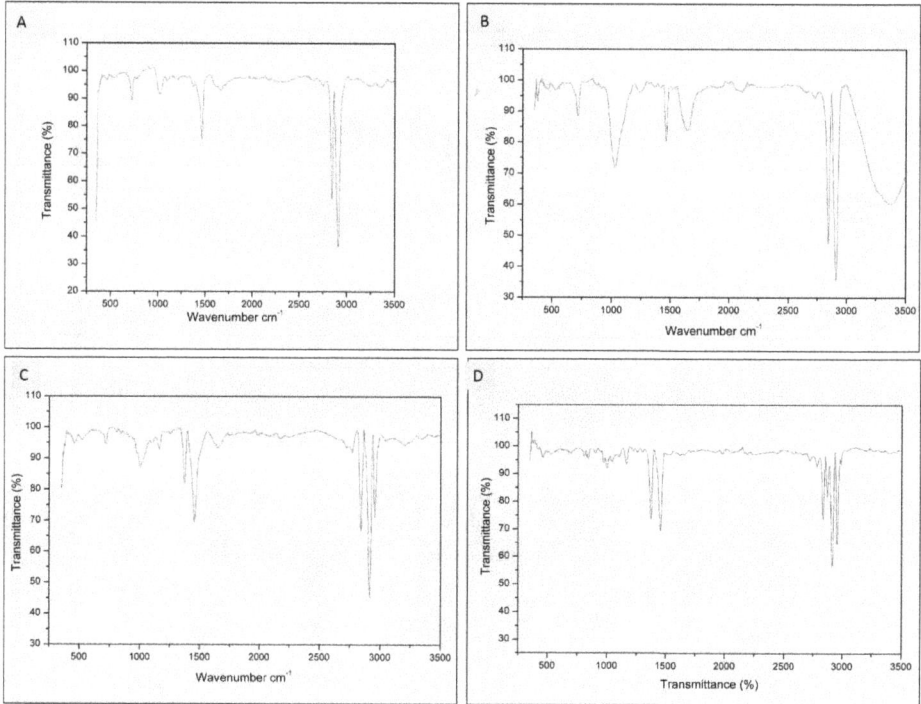

**Fig. 6.11** FTIR peaks of the microplastics (A- polyethylene; B- polypropylene, C & D- polystyrene)

*"A Study on the Persistent Pollutants and their Ecological Risk from Surface Sediments of Selected Estuaries, Kerala, SW Coast of India"*

Page | 143

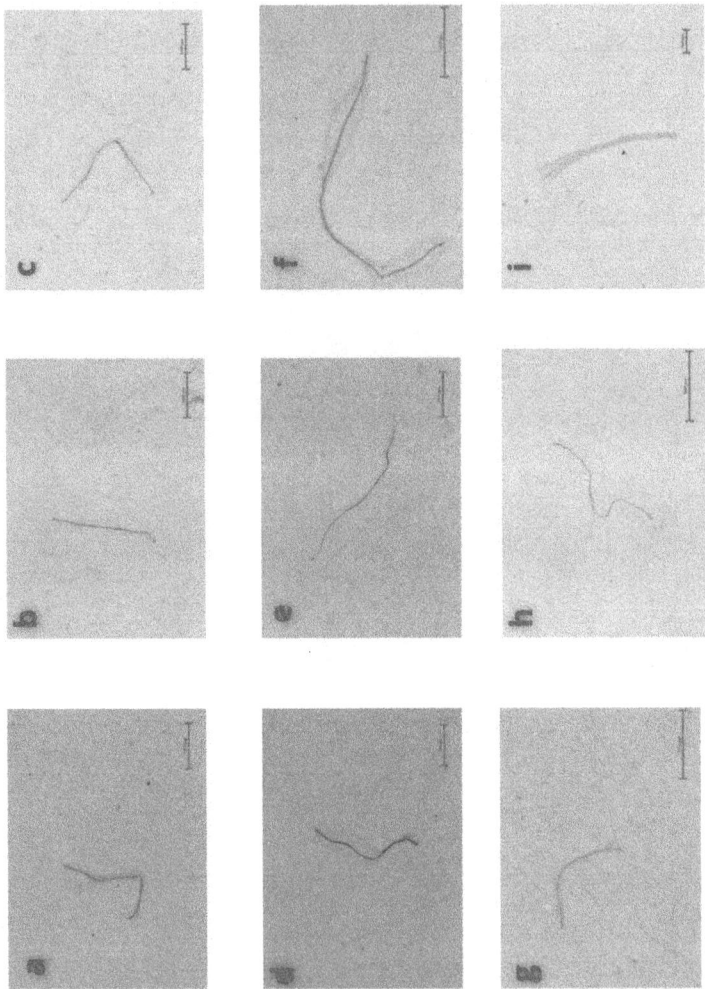

**Fig. 6.12** showing fibrous shape microplastics in the surface sediments of the selected estuaries in Kerala

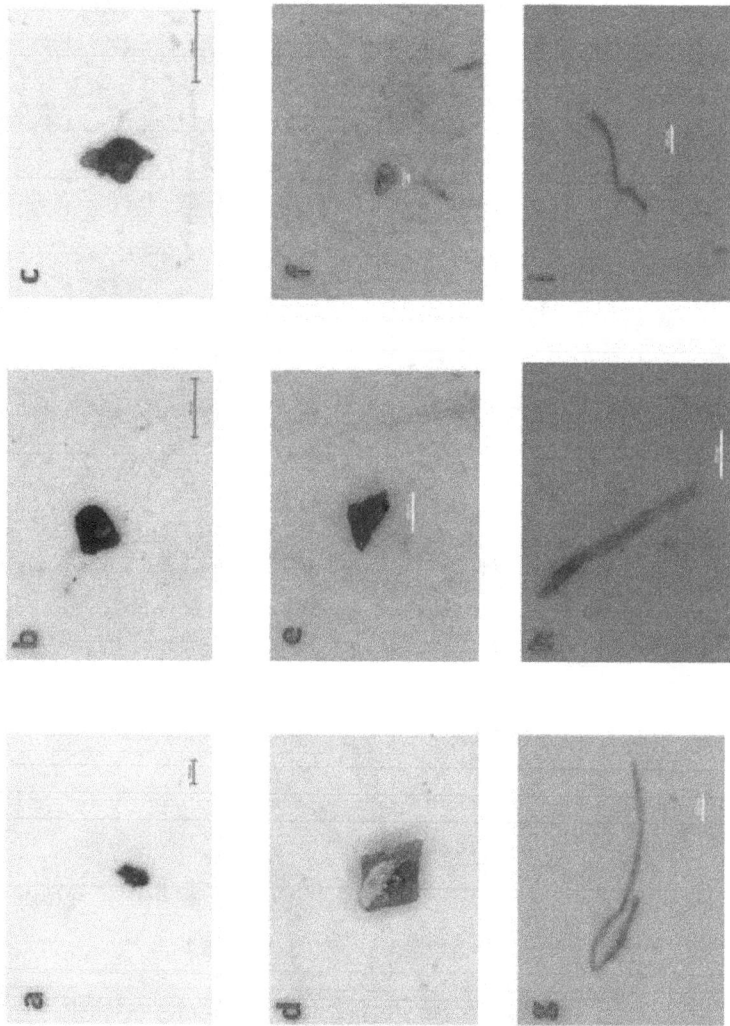

**Fig. 6.13** showing fragment (a – e) and filament (f – i) shape microplastics in the surface sediments of the selected estuaries in Kerala

**Table. 6.1** Representing various characteristic features of Microplastics in Kadinamkulam estuary, Kerala

| S.No | SHAPE | | | COMPOSITION | | | COLOUR | | SIZE (in µm) | | | Total |
|---|---|---|---|---|---|---|---|---|---|---|---|---|
| | Fibre | Fragment | Filament | Polyethylene | Polypropylene | Polyester | Colored Plastic | White Plastic | <1000 | 1000-3000 | >3000 | |
| 2 | 6 | 5 | 2 | 5 | 2 | 6 | 9 | 4 | 9 | 2 | 2 | 13 |
| 4 | 14 | 4 | 2 | 4 | 2 | 14 | 15 | 5 | 14 | 4 | 2 | 20 |
| 7 | 11 | 8 | 2 | 10 | | 11 | 19 | 2 | 17 | 3 | 1 | 21 |
| 9 | 7 | 9 | 1 | 9 | 1 | 7 | 12 | 5 | 15 | 0 | 2 | 17 |
| 12 | 8 | 10 | | 7 | 3 | 8 | 15 | 3 | 11 | 6 | 1 | 18 |
| 16 | 7 | 3 | | 3 | | 7 | 8 | 2 | 7 | 3 | 0 | 10 |
| 19 | 6 | 4 | 1 | 4 | 1 | 6 | 9 | 2 | 8 | 1 | 2 | 11 |
| 22 | 3 | 2 | 2 | 2 | 2 | 3 | 7 | | 6 | 0 | 1 | 7 |
| Avg | 7.75 | 5.62 | 1.66 | 5.5 | 1.8 | 7.75 | 11.75 | 3.29 | 10.88 | 2.38 | 1.38 | 14.63 |
| Min | 3 | 2 | 1 | 2 | 1 | 3 | 7 | 2 | 6 | 0 | 0 | 7 |
| Max | 14 | 10 | 2 | 10 | 3 | 14 | 19 | 5 | 17 | 6 | 2 | 21 |

**Table. 6.2** Representing various characteristic features of Microplastics in Anchuthengu estuary, Kerala

| S.No | SHAPE | | | COMPOSITION | | | COLOUR | | SIZE (in μm) | | | Total |
|------|-------|----------|----------|--------------|---------------|-----------|------------------|-----------------|-------|-----------|-------|-------|
|      | Fibre | Fragment | Filament | Polyethylene | Polypropylene | Polyester | Colored Plastic | White Plastic | <1000 | 1000-3000 | >3000 |       |
| 24   | 10    | 18       | 1        | 11           | 8             | 10        | 23               | 6               | 19    | 7         | 3     | 29    |
| 28   | 8     | 3        | 0        | 3            | 0             | 8         | 8                | 3               | 6     | 3         | 2     | 11    |
| 30   | 10    | 8        | 0        | 8            | 0             | 10        | 15               | 3               | 15    | 3         | 0     | 18    |
| 33   | 13    | 3        | 0        | 4            | 2             | 10        | 14               | 2               | 12    | 3         | 1     | 16    |
| 36   | 8     | 5        | 2        | 5            | 2             | 8         | 11               | 4               | 10    | 3         | 2     | 15    |
| 39   | 11    | 16       | 3        | 16           | 3             | 11        | 23               | 7               | 22    | 5         | 3     | 30    |
| 43   | 10    | 15       | 11       | 15           | 11            | 10        | 26               | 10              | 27    | 3         | 6     | 36    |
| 45   | 6     | 1        | 0        | 1            | 1             | 5         | 7                | 0               | 7     | 0         | 0     | 7     |
| 48   | 6     | 7        | 0        | 4            | 3             | 6         | 8                | 5               | 9     | 3         | 1     | 13    |
| 54   | 3     | 2        | 2        | 2            | 2             | 3         | 7                | 0               | 5     | 0         | 2     | 7     |
| **Avg** | **8.5** | **7.8** | **2.7** | **6.9** | **4** | **8.1** | **14.2** | **4** | **13.2** | **3** | **2** | **18.2** |
| **Min** | **3** | **1** | **0** | **1** | **1** | **3** | **7** | **0** | **5** | **0** | **0** | **7** |
| **Max** | **13** | **18** | **11** | **16** | **11** | **11** | **26** | **10** | **27** | **7** | **6** | **36** |

**Table. 6.3** Representing various characteristic features of Microplastics in Kappil - Hariharapuram estuary, Kerala

| S.No | SHAPE | | | COMPOSITION | | | COLOUR | | SIZE (in μm) | | | Total |
|---|---|---|---|---|---|---|---|---|---|---|---|---|
| | Fibre | Fragment | Filament | Polyethylene | Polypropylene | Polyester | Colored Plastic | White Plastic | <1000 | 1000-3000 | >3000 | |
| 56 | 0 | 6 | 1 | 6 | 1 | 0 | 5 | 2 | 4 | 2 | 1 | 7 |
| 60 | 13 | 9 | 0 | 7 | 2 | 13 | 16 | 6 | 16 | 5 | 1 | 22 |
| 64 | 13 | 3 | 2 | 1 | 2 | 15 | 15 | 3 | 15 | 3 | 0 | 18 |
| 66 | 16 | 2 | 1 | 1 | 3 | 15 | 15 | 4 | 13 | 4 | 2 | 19 |
| 71 | 8 | 4 | 0 | 4 | 0 | 8 | 9 | 3 | 8 | 2 | 2 | 12 |
| 75 | 0 | 6 | 0 | 6 | 0 | 0 | 5 | 1 | 3 | 2 | 1 | 6 |
| 76 | 7 | 3 | 1 | 3 | 1 | 7 | 8 | 3 | 7 | 3 | 1 | 11 |
| 77 | 2 | 1 | 0 | 0 | 1 | 2 | 3 | 0 | 2 | 1 | 0 | 3 |
| 81 | 0 | 7 | 3 | 7 | 3 | 0 | 8 | 2 | 8 | 1 | 1 | 10 |
| Avg | 8.42 | 4.37 | 1.75 | 4.14 | 2 | 10 | 9.88 | 2.75 | 9 | 2.63 | 1 | 12.63 |
| Min | 0 | 1 | 1 | 1 | 1 | 2 | 3 | 0 | 2 | 1 | 0 | 3 |
| Max | 16 | 9 | 3 | 7 | 3 | 15 | 16 | 6 | 16 | 5 | 2 | 22 |

**Table. 6.4** Representing various characteristic features of Microplastics in Kayamkulam estuary, Kerala

| S.No | SHAPE | | | COMPOSITION | | | COLOUR | | SIZE (in µm) | | | Total |
|---|---|---|---|---|---|---|---|---|---|---|---|---|
| | Fibre | Fragment | Filament | Polyethylene | Polypropylene | Polyester | Colored Plastic | White Plastic | <1000 | 1000-3000 | >3000 | |
| 83 | 6 | 8 | 0 | 2 | 8 | 4 | 13 | 1 | 6 | 7 | 1 | 14 |
| 84 | 3 | 0 | 0 | 1 | 0 | 2 | 1 | 2 | 1 | 1 | 1 | 3 |
| 86 | 4 | 0 | 0 | 1 | 0 | 3 | 4 | 0 | 1 | 3 | 0 | 4 |
| 88 | 4 | 1 | 1 | 2 | 2 | 2 | 6 | 0 | 5 | 1 | 0 | 6 |
| 90 | 9 | 1 | 0 | 3 | 1 | 6 | 9 | 1 | 7 | 3 | 0 | 10 |
| 92 | 23 | 7 | 0 | 9 | 7 | 14 | 23 | 7 | 20 | 8 | 2 | 30 |
| 96 | 1 | 0 | 0 | 0 | 0 | 1 | 1 | 0 | 1 | 0 | 0 | 1 |
| 97 | 7 | 10 | 2 | 2 | 10 | 7 | 10 | 9 | 13 | 5 | 1 | 19 |
| 98 | 12 | 2 | 0 | 4 | 2 | 8 | 2 | 12 | 11 | 3 | 0 | 14 |
| 99 | 4 | 30 | 0 | 1 | 30 | 3 | 2 | 32 | 27 | 5 | 2 | 34 |
| 101 | 2 | 8 | 0 | 1 | 8 | 1 | 0 | 10 | 7 | 3 | 0 | 10 |
| 103 | 37 | 5 | 2 | 15 | 5 | 24 | 22 | 22 | 21 | 16 | 7 | 44 |
| 106 | 6 | 1 | 2 | 3 | 1 | 5 | 7 | 2 | 5 | 4 | 0 | 9 |
| 108 | 6 | 0 | 0 | 2 | 0 | 4 | 6 | 0 | 3 | 2 | 1 | 6 |
| 109 | 8 | 0 | 2 | 3 | 0 | 7 | 10 | 0 | 6 | 3 | 1 | 10 |
| 110 | 0 | 0 | 1 | 0 | 0 | 1 | 1 | 0 | 1 | 0 | 0 | 1 |
| 111 | 4 | 2 | 0 | 1 | 2 | 3 | 6 | 0 | 4 | 2 | 0 | 6 |
| Avg | 8.00 | 4.41 | 0.59 | 2.94 | 4.47 | 5.59 | 7.24 | 5.76 | 8.18 | 3.88 | 0.94 | 13 |
| Min | 0 | 0 | 0 | 0 | 0 | 1 | 0 | 0 | 1 | 0 | 0 | 1 |
| Max | 37 | 30 | 2 | 15 | 30 | 24 | 23 | 32 | 27 | 16 | 7 | 44 |

## 6.7 THE COMPARATIVE RESULTS

The distribution of microplastics in estuarine surface sediments was shown and compared with other estuaries around the world (Table. 6.5). The comparative results of the other studies show that lowest distribution of microplastics except Pearl River estuary, China. Sruthy and Ramasamy (2017) have reported the distribution of microplastics in Vembanad estuary, southwest coast of India. This study clearly suggests that low density polyethylene is the most dominant type of polymer component of the MPs. The origin of the microplastic in the Vembanad Lake is most probably due to fragmentation of larger plastic debris and improper disposal of plastic debris. In the present investigation, the following descending order in the abundance of microplastic composition is observed: polyester (95 particles - 42.98%) > polypropylene (76 particles – 34.38%) > polyethylene (50 particles – 22.62%). The distribution of the microplastics in the estuarine sediments was significantly controlled by the sea water inundation in the estuary and distance of sampling points from the coast.

The present study reports the spatial variations in the number of microplastics, colour, shape, size and composition in the surface sediments of chosen estuaries, Kerala coast of India. The mean abundance of the microplastic distribution in the sediments of selected estuaries was 628 particles/kg. The occurrence of the microplastic in sediments was due to the proximity of urban regions, distance of the sampling point from the coast. The FTIR studies revealed that polyethylene, polyester and polypropylene were the dominant polymers among the different types of microplastics in estuarine surface sediments. The proper solid waste management, adoption of correct policies and creation of the awareness among the people the negative impact of microplastics to the environment may be the solution for this problem.

**Table. 6.5** A comparative investigation on the distribution of microplastics in different estuaries around the world

| S.No | Studied Estuaries | Location | Microplastics in sediments | References |
|------|-------------------|----------|----------------------------|------------|
| 1 | Liaohe Estuary | China | 120±46 (particles/ d.w. Kg) | Xu et al., 2020 |
| 2 | Yondingxinhe Estuary | China | 85.0±40.1 (particles/ d.w. Kg) | Wu et al., 2019 |
| 3 | Haihe Estuary | China | 216.1±92.1 (particles/ d.w. Kg) | Wu et al., 2019 |
| 4 | Changjiang Estuary | China | 121±9 (particles/ d.w. Kg) | Peng et al., 2017 |
| 5 | Gunabara Bay | Brazil | 528±30 (particles/ d.w. Kg) | Alves and Figueiredo, 2019 |
| 6 | Tampa bay | U.S.A | 280 (particles/ d.w. Kg) | McEachern et al., 2019 |
| 7 | Jagir Estuary | Indonesia | 92-590 (particles/ d.w. Kg) | Firdaus et al., 2020 |
| 8 | Warnow Estuary | Germany | 46-100 (particles/ d.w. Kg) | Enders et al., 2019 |
| 9 | Yangtze Estuary | China | 110-60 (particles/ d.w. Kg) | Li et al., 2020 |
| 10 | Pearl River Estuary | Hongkong | 5595±27417 (particles m$^{-2}$) | Fok and Cheung, 2015 |
| 11 | Vembanad Lake | India | 252.8 (particles m$^{-2}$) | Sruthy and Ramasamy, 2017 |
| 12 | Winyah Bay | U.S.A | 221±25.6 (particles m$^{-2}$) | Gray et al., 2018 |
| 13 | Charleston Harbor | U.S.A | 413.8±76.7 (particles m$^{-2}$) | Gray et al., 2018 |
| 15 | Selected estuaries, Kerala | India | 628 particles/kg. | Present study |

## 6.8 RISK ASSESSMENT OF MPs IN SEDIMENTS

Microplastics along the additives often known as cocktail of contaminants, persistent organic pollutants and heavy metals exist in the environment (Rochman, 2015). The mixture of microplastics with its additives can be bioavailable to numerous biota and humans through ingestion (Hartmann *et al.*, 2017). As a result, it's critical to analyse the ecotoxicological risk of MPs in order to have a clear picture of the potential harm when they're consumed by biota. Chakraborty *et al.* (2014) explained due to rapid industrialization, climatic changes and persistent pollutants began to contaminate estuarine sediments through multiple pathways resulted in association with several health issues to various biota along the coast for the past few decades in India. For the past three years, the abundance and chemical composition of MPs in diverse environmental matrices have been closely examined in India (Veerasingam *et al.*, 2020). Many marine and terrestrial organisms ingest MPs which may transfer well into the human food chain (Naidu, 2019; Kumar *et al.*, 2018 and Daniel *et al.*, 2020), leading to the adverse health issues to biota and humans as well (Pan *et al.*, 2021). Unreacted monomers and hazardous additives remain while synthesizing the MPs from a chain of monomers by polymerization process. Due to photo degradation and thermo degradation, MPs in sea surface and beach releases hazardous additives. The United Nations' Globally Harmonized System of classification and cataloguing of chemicals categorizes plastics with chemical ingredients greater than 50% are ranked as hazardous (Lithner *et al.*, 2011; Rochman *et al.*, 2013). Results based on the ecological risk assessment of MPs in the sediments have not received much attention. Using Polymer Hazard Index (PHI) and Potential Ecological Risk Index (PERI) as the parameters, the ecological risk assessment of MPs in estuarine, marine and terrestrial sediments is assessed.

## 6.9 MICROPLASTICS POLLUSION INDICES

### 6.9.1 Polymer Hazard Index (PHI)

To assess the possible dangers of MPs in surface sediments, we looked at both their concentration and chemical composition (Xu *et al.*, 2018). To estimate the ecological harm, chemical toxicity of various polymer types of MPs is considered (Lithner *et al.*, 2011). The polymer hazard assessment of MPs was calculated using the following formula:

$$PHI = \Sigma Pn \times Sn$$

where, Pn is the fraction of specified polymer types (Table. 6.6) recovered at each sampling point, and Sn is the hazard scores of polymer types of MPs determined from Lithner et al (2011).

### 6.9.2 Potential Ecological Risk Index (PERI)

The Potential Ecological Risk Index (PERI) is used to determine the extent of MPs contamination in sediments (Peng et al., 2018). The equations used to calculate the PERI are as follows:

$$Cif = Ci/Cin$$
$$Ti\ r = \Sigma^n_{n=1}\ Pn\ /Ci \times Sn$$
$$Eir = Tir \times Cif$$

where, Ci is the concentration of pollutant 'i' (i.e., microplastic) and Cin is the concentration of unpolluted samples. Toxicity and biological sensitivity are represented by the toxicity coefficient (Tir). The toxicity coefficient is calculated by multiplying the percentage of particular polymers in the entire sample (Pn/Ci) by the plastic polymer hazard score (Sn).

**Table. 6.6** Representing the various Hazard score based on MPs

| PHI | Hazard category | PERI | Risk category |
|---|---|---|---|
| 0-1 | I | <150 | Minor |
| 1-10 | II | 150-300 | Medium |
| 10-100 | III | 300-600 | High |
| 100-1000 | IV | 600-1220 | Danger |
| >1000 | V | >1200 | Extreme |

**Table. 6.7** Representing pollution indices of Microplastics from selective estuaries in Kerala

| KADINAMKULAM | | |
|---|---|---|
| S.No | PHI | PERI |
| 2 | 1823.08 | 7900.00 |
| 4 | 2330.00 | 15533.33 |
| 7 | 2095.24 | 14666.67 |
| 9 | 1823.53 | 10333.33 |
| 12 | 1777.78 | 10666.67 |
| 16 | 2430.00 | 8100.00 |
| 19 | 2045.45 | 7500.00 |
| 22 | 1628.57 | 3800.00 |
| Avg | 1994.21 | 9812.50 |
| Min | 1628.57 | 3800.00 |
| Max | 2430.00 | 15533.33 |

| ANCHUTHENGU | | |
|---|---|---|
| S.No | PHI | PERI |
| 24 | 1479.31 | 14300.00 |
| 28 | 2481.82 | 9100.00 |
| 30 | 2155.56 | 12933.33 |
| 33 | 2162.50 | 11533.33 |
| 36 | 1980.00 | 9900.00 |
| 39 | 1696.67 | 16966.67 |
| 43 | 1322.22 | 15866.67 |
| 45 | 2314.29 | 5400.00 |
| 48 | 1746.15 | 7566.67 |
| 54 | 1628.57 | 3800.00 |
| Avg | 1896.71 | 10736.67 |
| Min | 1322.22 | 3800.00 |
| Max | 2481.82 | 16966.67 |

| KAPPIL- HARIHARAPURAM | | |
|---|---|---|
| S.No | PHI | PERI |
| 56 | 957.14 | 2233.33 |
| 60 | 2131.82 | 15633.33 |
| 64 | 2572.22 | 15433.33 |
| 66 | 2442.11 | 15466.67 |
| 71 | 2366.67 | 9466.67 |
| 75 | 1100.00 | 2200.00 |
| 76 | 2218.18 | 8133.33 |
| 77 | 2033.33 | 2033.33 |
| 81 | 800.00 | 2666.67 |
| Avg | 1958.04 | 8879.17 |
| Min | 800.00 | 2033.33 |
| Max | 2572.22 | 15633.33 |

| KAYAMKULAM | | |
|---|---|---|
| S.No | PHI | PERI |
| 83 | 1071.42 | 15000 |
| 84 | 2366.66 | 7100 |
| 86 | 2525 | 10100 |
| 88 | 1400 | 8400 |
| 90 | 2140 | 21400 |
| 92 | 1753.33 | 52600 |
| 96 | 3000 | 3000 |
| 97 | 1273.68 | 24200 |
| 98 | 2042.85 | 28600 |
| 99 | 385.29 | 13100 |
| 101 | 490 | 4900 |
| 103 | 2022.72 | 89000 |
| 106 | 2044.44 | 18400 |
| 108 | 2366.66 | 14200 |
| 109 | 2430 | 24300 |
| 110 | 3000 | 3000 |
| 111 | 1716.66 | 10300 |
| Avg | 1884.04 | 20447.06 |
| Min | 385.29 | 3000 |
| Max | 3000 | 89000 |

The overall risk of MPs pollution in present study was categorized as Hazard level IV to V, based on PHI values (Table. 6.6 and Table. 6.7). Due to the existence of MPs with high hazard scores such as PA and PS, the PHI values of Kadinamkulam are high (>1000). In Kappil-Hariharapuram (S. no. 56), (S.no. 81) two samples and Kayamkulam estuary two samples (S.no. 99 and 101) have values lesser than 1000 falling under PHI category IV, respectively. Apart from these four samples, all the other samples in the analyzed estuarine sediments falling under the PHI category V (Table. 6.6). Although the hazard scores of PP and PE are smaller than those of PS, they should not be overlooked when evaluating the risk. Furthermore, even though the MP concentration is low, the chemical toxicity of the substance should not be overlooked.

The potential ecological risk index (PERI) values of selected estuarine sediments of the present study show extreme ecological risk (PERI: >1200) from collective MP polymers in sediments from Kadinamkulam, Anchuthengu, Kappil- Hariharapuram and Kayamkulam. The hazard score is used to calculate the PERI, and since the toxicity score for PS is high, and that caused the higher values of PERI. Although there is no discernible relationship between MP abundance and PHI based on the insights gathered, increasing MP abundance may pose an ecological risk. The combined utilisation of PHI and PERI in this work offered a baseline ecological risk assessment induced by MP contamination in selected estuarine sediments along Kerala's south coast.

Department of Geology, UNOM

# CHAPTER-VII

# SOURCE AND DISTRIBUTION OF POLYCYCLIC AROMATIC HYDROCARBONS IN SEDIMENTS

## 7.1 INTRODUCTION

Polycyclic aromatic hydrocarbons (PAHs) have been identified as significant carcinogens, mutagens, and ubiquitous contaminants in a number of media, including air, food, sediments, and water, according to numerous studies. To solve components of interest from solid samples such as soil or sediments using a suitable solvent, a variety of solid-liquid extraction (SLE) procedures were applied. Maceration, ultrasonic-assisted extraction (UAE), microwave-assisted extraction (MAE), Soxhlet extraction (SE), and accelerated solvent extraction (ASE) were used to extract this compound from selected environmental samples (Ghassempour *et al.,* 2008; Madej *et al.,* 2018). The extraction approach was chosen based on a number of variables, including capital and operating costs, ease of operation, the amount of organic solvent required, and the availability of a standardised method (Dean *et al.,* 1997). The US Environmental Protection Agency (US EPA) recommends the soxhlet extraction process for extracting semi-volatile and non-volatile organics from solid matrices. They are, however, time-consuming techniques that require a lot of solvent and aren't suited for separating thermally degradable chemicals (De Castro *et al.,* 1998).

The ultrasonic probe extraction procedure is a useful technique because of its high extraction efficiency, low equipment costs, convenience of use, lack of sample preparation, lower extraction temperatures, and applicability for trace organic chemicals in soil and sediments (Song *et al.,* 2002; Banjoo *et al.,* 2005). The efficiency of this approach, however, is affected by the solvent or solvent composition, extraction time, sample load, and water content (Berset *et al.,* 1999). Acetone was shown to be the most efficient solvent for extracting the US EPA's 16 priority pollutant PAHs in soils, according to Sun *et al.,* 1998. During oven drying of samples at 45° C, about 16 percent of the hydrocarbon components were lost (Wong, 1980; Berset *et al.,* 1999). Ramzi *et al.* (2017), published a remarkable comprehensive investigation on the dynamics of polycyclic aromatic hydrocarbons (PAHs) in surface sediments at the Cochin estuary. The goal of this study is to determine the concentrations of 16 USEPA-listed PAHs in surface sediments from selected estuaries on Kerala's west coast.

### 7.2. SAMPLING AND PRE-TREATMENT PROCESS

Twenty surface sediments were collected from three selected estuaries of the Kerala coast (Kayamkulam, Anchuthengu, Kadinamkulam, and Varkala-Hariharapuram estuaries). Using a pre-clean stainless-steel spatula, the surface sediment was transferred to amber-colored glass jars and stored in the ice box (Fig. 7.1). The sediments were immediately transferred to the laboratory and stored in a deep freezer at -20°C until they were analysed.

### 7.3 SEPARATION AND ANALYSIS OF PAHs

During the extraction of the PAH fraction, the sonication/ultrasonic agitation method was applied to achieve greater extraction efficiencies (Sun *et al.,* 1998). As a result, the freeze-dried and homogenised sediment was utilised to extract the PAH using a dichloromethane – methanol (2:1) solvent mixture in a sonication/ultrasonic agitation bath for 48 hours, and the resulting extract was treated with activated granular copper to remove sulphur impurities. Finally, the extract was purified using the silica-alumina (2:1) column cleanup method after the extracted solution was evaporated using the rotary evaporation method. The aliphatic compounds were then removed from the column by eluting it with n-hexane. The column was then eluted with n-hexane to remove the aliphatic compounds, followed by a combination of n-hexane and dichloromethane to remove the PAH compounds (3:7 ratio). The near-dryness extract was prepared for PAH detection using 500 µl n-hexane after the final extract was evaporated by a moderate nitrogen stream. A flame ionisation detector on an Agilent 7890B Series Gas Chromatograph was used to evaluate sixteen PAHs listed by the USEPA. The temperature of the column for analyses was set to 60°C (starting time, 2 minutes) at a rate of 10°C per minute, then to 120–300°C at a rate of 3° C per minute, and finally to 310° C for 5 minutes. During both injection modes, the injector and detector were kept at 280° C and 325° C, respectively, and the injection volume was 2 L. On the basis of the recovery output of a known amount of PAH reference combination, the extraction efficiency was double-checked. PAH recovery rates ranged from 82 percent to 95 percent. All chemical analyses were performed in triplicate, and the output values were represented in dry weight.

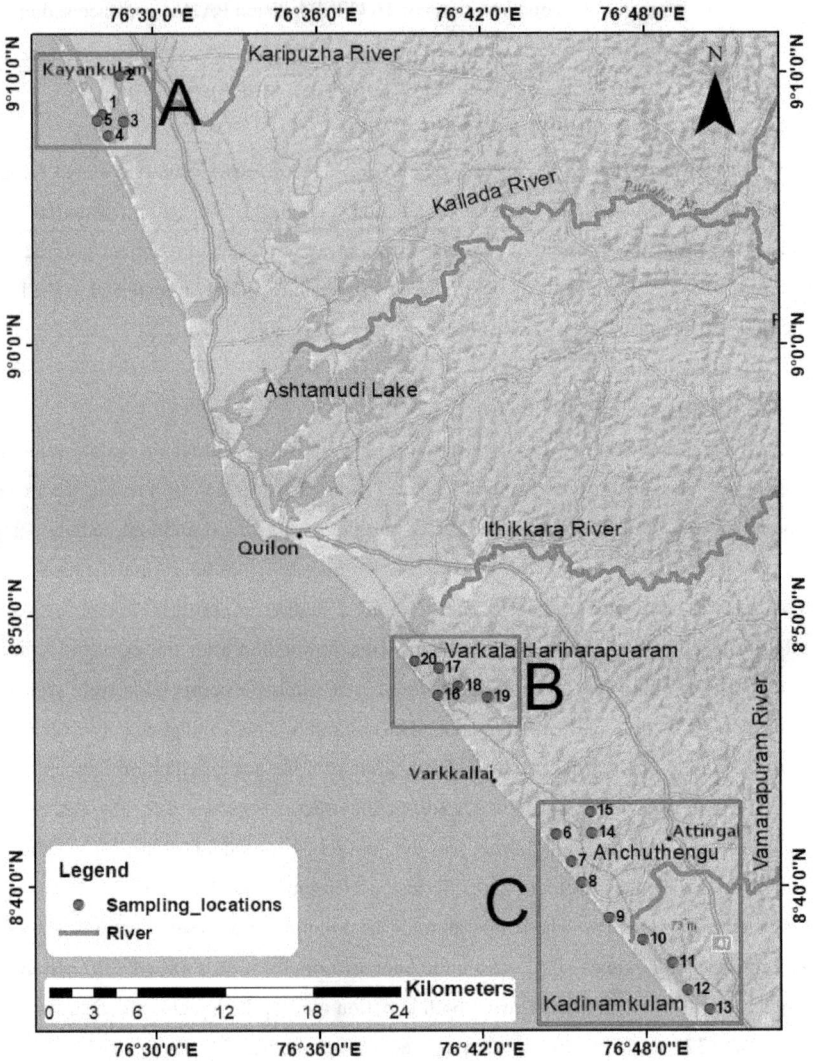

**Fig. 7.1** sampling locations for the PAHs analysis of the selected estuaries of Kerala, Southwest coast of India

## 7.4 CONCENTRATION OF LMW AND HMW RING PAHs

Low molecular weight PAHs (2 and 3 rings) and high molecular weight PAHs (2 and 3 rings) were used to classify the PAH fractions examined (4 and above rings). Table. 7.1 lists the names of the PAH fractions tested, as well as their number of rings, concentration range, mean, standard deviation, Toxic Effects-Range Low (ERL), Toxic Effects-Range Medium (ERM), Carcinogenic potency, and molecular weight. The fine-grained silt to clay grade sediment fractions dominated the surface sediments of the estuaries, and only a few samples from the mouths of the estuaries were sandy. With a mean value of 15.08 ng/g, total PAH concentrations vary from 0.47 to 126.64 ng/g. The concentration of low molecular weight rings (LMW rings - 2 & 3 rings) in the sediments ranges from 0 to 5.42 ng/g, whereas the concentration of heavy molecular weight rings (HMW rings - 4 & above rings) ranges from 5.42 to 122.1 ng/g. HMW-PAHs enriched the estuary sediments, accounting for roughly 93.76 percent of the overall concentration, followed by LMW-PAHs (LMW-PAH – 6.23 percent). Naphthalene, Acenaphthene, and Anthracene were found to be highly enriched among the LMW ring PAHs, whereas Benzo(b)fluoranthene, Benzo(k)fluoranthene, Benzo(a)pyrene, Indeno[1,2,3-cd] pyrene, and Benz[ghi]perylene were found to be highly concentrated among the HMW-PAHs (Table. 7.1). In the inner section of the estuary, especially in Anchuthengu and Kadinamkulam estuaries, the sediment-associated 16 PAHs distribution was higher. Similar studies on the Cochin estuary found that the distance between the sampling point and the estuary mouth, as well as inundated sea water, influences the dispersion of PAHs. Sediment features, fluvial and tidal flow mechanisms all had an indirect impact on PAH enrichment in the inner estuarine system. Benzo[a]pyrene is one of the most dangerous of the parent PAHs, and it is employed as a surrogate chemical marker for genotoxic organic chemicals, according to Safe, 1998. The PAHs may have come from nearby anthropogenic activities such as road run-off and/or combusted particles from automobiles, or possibly from railway tracks (Vane *et al.,* 2020). According to earlier research, the interaction between organic carbon/natural organic materials, such as humic substance coasting on the mineral surface, has a direct impact on PAH distribution (Stout and Emsbo-Mattingly, 2008; Ukalska Jaruga *et al.,* 2019). Furthermore, this research reveals that the link between TOC and PAHs in sediment cores has a positive association. The Mersey estuary (Vane et al., 2007) showed a negative association between grain size (sand-silt-clay ratio), whereas PAHs in sediment and pore water of the Yellow

River China showed a positive link with silt and fine grain fractions. This study's surface sediments reveal a similar finding, particularly in the inner parts of estuaries where the sediment is richer with fine fractions (Yu *et al.,* 2009; Maruya *et al.,* 1997).

PAHs entered the marine environment via high-temperature pyrolytic processes as well as a petrogenic source (Xu *et al.,* 2007). Monsoonal shifts, land/river runoff, and the combustion of pyrolytic source materials all played a role in the rapid growth of PAHs in the Cochin estuary. In addition, the overall PAH concentration in the Cochin estuary was found to be 100 times greater than in the current study. A study of PAHs in sediments was compared to earlier examinations from India and around the world. Sediment texture, organic content, and flow parameters were all found to have a major impact on PAH distribution in aquatic environments in previous research (He *et al.,* 2014). The concentration of PAHs in selected estuaries of the west coast was lower than in the other study region (Table. 7.2).

PAHs in sediments have been linked to delayed hatching, induction of deformities, disruption of larvae swimming activity, and DNA damage in bottom-dwelling fish (Malins *et al.,* 1988; Vethaak and Rheinalt, 1992, Cousin and Cachot, 2014). PAH sources can be identified using the ratio of low molecular weight to high molecular weight PAH components. The estimated ratio greater than 1 denotes a petrogenic source of PAH, whereas the ratio less than 1 denotes a pyrolytic source. The ratio of LMW/HMW PAHs in this study indicates that pyrolytic fractions predominate in these estuaries.

NOAA sediment quality guidelines have been widely used to determine PAH contamination levels in water systems "NOAA, 1999". Long *et al.* (1995) proposed two important tools, such as Effect Range Low (ERL) and Effect Range Median (ERM), to determine the quality level of sediments. Both indicators (ERL and ERM) helped to list thresholds and rare biological adverse effects. Toxicological values are used with their active areas to assess the quality of the sediments., 10th percentile is classified as the ERL and the 50th percentile is classified as the ERM (Long *et al.,* 1995). The PAH distribution at the selected Kerala estuary indicates that the PAH concentration was lower than the ERL and ERM values proposed by SQGs. The PAH analysis results conclude that the superficial sediment deposits of the selected estuary system fall into the low pollution and low risk categories.

The total amount of potentially carcinogenic PAH congers in the sediment was used to determine its toxicity range (TCPAH - BaA, Chr, BbF, BkF, BaP, DbA, and InP fractions; Chen and Chen, 2011). The TCPAH levels in the estuarine surface sediments ranged from 16 to 44.21 ng/g. The TCPAH analytical result was lower than the ERL-ERM levels reported by SQGs (1373–8410 ng/g; Long *et al.*, 1995). The toxic equivalent (TEQ) of each PAH was calculated using the equation below (Nasher *et al.*, 2013; Li *et al.*, 2015).

$$Total\ TEQ = \sum_i Ci \times TEFi$$

TEFi is the toxicity factor of specific individual fractions, and C i is the concentration of an individual PAH fraction. BaA, Ch, BbF, BkF, BaP, IP, and DbA have TEFs of 0.1, 0.001, 0.1, 0.01, 1, 0.1, and 1. (USEPA, 1993). The overall TEQ value premeditated fluctuated from 0.20 to 54.80 ng/g (Fig. 7. 2 and Table. 7.3). A comparison of TEQ values from other research zones shows that the TEQ obtained in this study was lower than in other parts of India and the world (Table. 7.4).

In comparison to other study regions across the world, the findings suggest that the surface sediments of selected estuaries along the Kerala coast were less contaminated. Furthermore, the current study region was less polluted by polycyclic aromatic hydrocarbons (PAHs) and posed less of an environmental danger.

**Table. 7.1** Concentration ranges, mean and standard deviation (S.D) of individual PAHs (ng/g) in the surface sediments,

Kayals of West coast of Kerala, India

| S.no | Name of the PAH | No of rings | Sediment (n = 20) | | | ERL | ERM | Carcinogenic potency[a] | Molecular weight |
|---|---|---|---|---|---|---|---|---|---|
| | | | Range (ng/g) | Mean (ng/g) | S.D. (ng/g) | | | | |
| 1 | Naphthalene (Nap) | 2-Ring | ND - 3.99 | 0.511 | 0.987 | 160 | 2100 | D | 128.18 |
| 2 | Acenaphthylene (Acy) | 3-Ring | ND | ND | ND | 44 | 640 | - | 152.2 |
| 3 | Acenaphthene (Ace) | 3-Ring | ND | ND | ND | 16 | 500 | - | 154.2 |
| 4 | Anthracene (Ant) | 3-Ring | ND - 2.12 | 0.106 | 0.474 | 853 | 1100 | D | 178.24 |
| 5 | Phenanthrene (Phe) | 3-Ring | ND - 2.15 | 0.250 | 0.579 | 240 | 1500 | D | 178.24 |
| 6 | Fluorene (Fl) | 3-Ring | ND - 0.55 | 0.028 | 0.123 | 19 | 540 | D | 166.23 |
| 7 | Benzo(a)anthracene (BaA) | 4-Ring | ND - 7.29 | 1.160 | 1.691 | 261 | 1600 | $B_2$ | 228.3 |
| 8 | Chrysene (Chr) | 4-Ring | ND - 6.88 | 0.800 | 1.559 | 384 | 2800 | $B_2$ | 228.3 |
| 9 | Fluoranthene (Flu) | 4-Ring | ND - 6.5 | 0.823 | 1.442 | 600 | 5100 | D | 202.26 |
| 10 | Pyrene (Pyr) | 4-Ring | ND - 6.71 | 0.763 | 1.492 | 665 | 2600 | D | 202.26 |
| 11 | Benzo(b)fluoranthene (BbF) | 5-Ring | ND - 12.19 | 1.727 | 2.692 | 320 | 1800 | $B_2$ | 252.32 |
| 12 | Benzo(k)fluoranthene (BkF) | 5-Ring | ND - 19.7 | 1.908 | 4.405 | 280 | 1620 | $B_2$ | 252.32 |
| 13 | Benzo(a)pyrene (BaP) | 5-Ring | ND - 21.28 | 2.211 | 4.645 | 430 | 1600 | $B_2$ | 252.32 |
| 14 | Dibenzo(a,h)anthracene (DBA) | 5-Ring | ND - 8.68 | 0.874 | 1.974 | 63.4 | 260 | $B_2$ | 278.35 |
| 15 | Indeno [1,2,3-cd] pyrene (InP) | 6-Ring | ND - 15.46 | 2.098 | 3.409 | - | - | $B_2$ | 276.34 |
| 16 | Benz[ghi]perylene | 6-Ring | ND - 17.41 | 1.074 | 3.951 | 430 | 1600 | D | 276.34 |

$B_2$ Probable carcinogen, D - not classifiable as to human carcinogenicity (USEPA carcinogenic classification[a]), S.D – Standard Deviation, ND –

Not detected, ERL - Toxic Effects-Range Low, ERM - Toxic Effects-Range Medium

**Table. 7.2** Comparison table of polycyclic aromatic hydrocarbon (PAHs) in the present study and other worldwide estuarine and coastal systems report

| S.no | Details of the study region | Concentration Sum of PAH | References |
|---|---|---|---|
| 1 | Mersey Estuary, UK | 626–3766 | Vane et al., 2007 |
| 2 | Norwegian harbors, Norway | 2100–31100 | Cornelissen et al., 2006 |
| 3 | Tokyo Bay, Japan | 534–292370 | Zakaria et al., 2002 |
| 4 | Yellow River, China | 464–2621 | Yu et al., 2009 |
| 5 | Himalayan lakes, Nepal | $67.9 \pm 22.1$ | Guzzella et al., 2011 |
| 6 | Seine River basin, France | 5000 - 90,000 | Lorgeoux et al., 2016 |
| 7 | Minnesota lakes, USA | $489.3 \pm 980.5$ | Crane, 2017 |
| 8 | Cochin estuary, India | 194–14149 | Ramzi et al., 2017 |
| 9 | Chitrapuzha River, India | 5046–33087 | Sanil Kumar et al., 2016 |
| 10 | Hugli river, India | 0–1839 | Zuloaga et al., 2013 |
| 11 | Iko River estuary mangrove system, Nigeria | 6100–35,270 | Essien et al., 2011 |
| 12 | Esterode Urias, estuary, Mexico | 27–418 | Jaward et al., 2012 |
| 13 | Patos Lagoon Estuary, Brazil | 89–10451 | Garcia et al., 2010 |
| 14 | Galician estuaries, NW Spain | 44–7901 | Perez-Fernandez et al., 2015 |
| 15 | Selangor River estuary, Malaysia | 203–964 | Masood et al., 2016 |
| 16 | Selected estuaries of west coast of Kerala | | Present study |

**Table. 7.3** Sample wise distribution of sand, silt and clay (in %), low molecular and high molecular weight rings (ng/g), Total PAH (ng/g) of surface sediments, Kayals of West coast of Kerala, India

| Location | 1 | 2 | 3 | 4 | 5 | 6 | 7 | 8 | 9 | 10 | 11 | 12 | 13 | 14 | 15 | 16 | 17 | 18 | 19 | 20 |
|---|---|---|---|---|---|---|---|---|---|---|---|---|---|---|---|---|---|---|---|---|
| Sand % | 73 | 18.2 | 73.8 | 23.6 | 96.6 | 69.6 | 86.2 | 29.4 | 83.4 | 75.2 | 13.8 | 4.2 | 85.8 | 4.6 | 2 | 42 | 2.2 | 0.8 | 44.4 | 94.4 |
| Silt % | 26.2 | 80.8 | 25.4 | 76 | 3 | 25.4 | 13.4 | 70.4 | 16.4 | 24.8 | 85.8 | 95.4 | 14 | 95 | 97.6 | 57.6 | 97 | 98.8 | 55 | 5.2 |
| Clay % | 0.8 | 1 | 0.8 | 0.4 | 0.4 | 5 | 0.4 | 0.2 | 0.2 | 0 | 0.4 | 0.4 | 0.2 | 0.4 | 0.4 | 0.4 | 0.8 | 0.4 | 0.6 | 0.4 |
| LMW rings | 0 | 0.81 | 5.42 | 2.77 | 0 | 0 | 0 | 0 | 0 | 0.65 | 0 | 0 | 1.28 | 4.54 | 1.05 | 0 | 0 | 0 | 1.35 | 0 |
| HMW rings | 1.38 | 10.16 | 11.14 | 7.56 | 0.47 | 0.8 | 1.94 | 12.68 | 3.34 | 5.68 | 19.73 | 3.33 | 27.68 | 122.1 | 8.12 | 0.51 | 3.06 | 0 | 13.83 | 15.18 |
| Total PAH | 1.38 | 10.97 | 16.56 | 10.33 | 0.47 | 0.8 | 1.94 | 12.68 | 3.34 | 6.33 | 19.73 | 3.33 | 28.96 | 126.64 | 9.17 | 0.51 | 3.06 | ND | 15.18 | 15.18 |
| Total TEQ | 0.60 | 4.75 | 7.17 | 4.47 | 0.20 | 0.35 | 0.84 | 5.49 | 1.45 | 2.74 | 8.54 | 1.44 | 12.53 | 54.80 | 3.97 | 0.22 | 1.32 | 0.00 | 6.57 | 6.57 |

ND – Not detected, LMW rings  - Low molecular weight rings (2 & 3 rings); HMW rings - High molecular weight rings (4 & above rings), TEQ – Toxic equivalent

**Table. 7.4** Comparison of TEQ values of surface sediments of the selected estuaries of Kerala coast, Southwest coast of India with data from other areas worldwide

| Study area | TEQ (ng/g) | References |
|---|---|---|
| Naples Harbour, Italy | 2–4723 | Sprovieri *et al.*, 2007 |
| Kaohsiung Harbor, Taiwan | 1404–1964 | Chen and Chen, 2011 |
| Bahia Blanca Estuary, Argentina | 0–1969 | Oliva *et al.*, 2015 |
| Meiliang Bay in China | 94–856 | Qiao *et al.*, 2006 |
| Xiamen Bay, China | 15–282 | Li *et al.*, 2010 |
| Ría Arousa, Spain | 1.2–820 | Perez-Fernandez *et al.*, 2015 |
| Sundarban mangrove wetland, Bangladesh | 13–1014 | Zuloaga *et al.*, 2013 |
| Sundarban mangrove wetland, India | 1–2451 | Zuloaga *et al.*, 2013 |
| West coastal of the Gulf of Tunis, Tunisia | 8–666.4 | Mzoughi and Chouba, 2011 |
| Cochin Estuary, India | 1–971 | Ramzi *et al.*, 2017 |
| Selected estuaries of Kerala Southwest coast of India | 0.29 – 54.80 | Present study |

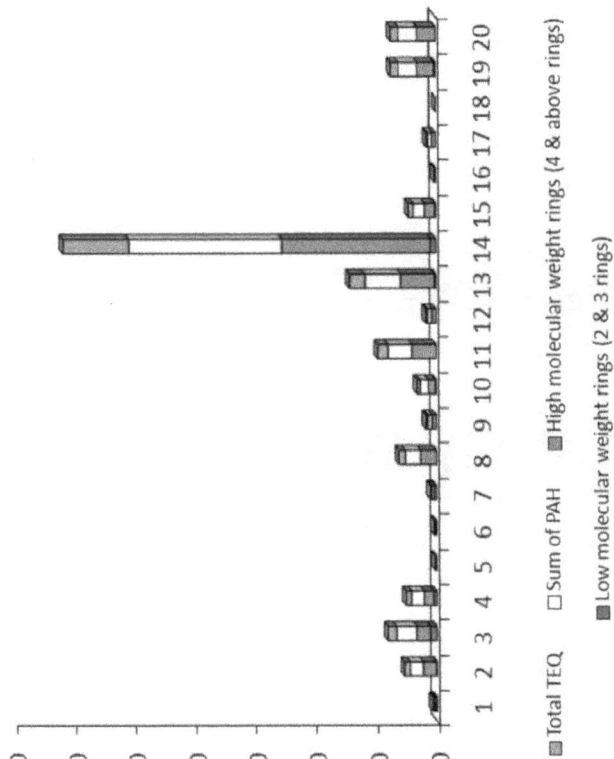

**Fig. 7. 2** Distribution of total TEQ, Sum of PAH, low and high molecular weight ring PAHs in the surface sediments, selected estuaries of Kerala, Southwest coast of India

# CHAPTER - VIII
# SUMMARY AND CONCLUSIONS

A total of 111 surface sediments from estuaries of southwest Kerala coast (Kadinamkulam - 23 samples; Anchuthengu - 32 samples; Kappil and Hariharapuram - 27 samples; Kayamkulam - 29 samples) were collected to analyse environmental parameters and the trace element geochemistry, out of which 44 sediment samples were chosen for the microplastics study and 20 sediment samples were selected for PAHs analysis. All these proxies were combined to enumerate the ecological risk caused by them to the environment.

## 8.1 TEXTURAL CHARACTERISTICS AND DEPOSITIONAL ENVIRONMENTS

Silt, sandy-silt and sand were the main sediment substrate in the selected estuaries. Silt is the dominant sediment observed in the estuary. Silty sediments deposit under calm waters and where the currents are weaker. The coarser sediments were deposited first at the estuarine mouth and the lower reaches of the river due to the density. Whereas at the zone of mixing, fine silt dominates as a result of decrease in the flow velocity of the stream and flocculation from intermixing water masses. From the observations the higher proportion of sand is a result of wave and tide-controlled sedimentation in the estuarine mouth and the fresh water influx.

Calcium carbonate is generally known as a dilutor of trace metal concentration and is contributed mainly by terrestrial run off and shelled organisms in water column. Calcium carbonate content in this study area shows a lot of variations. In Kadinamkulam the calcium carbonate percentage in the surface sediments varies from 0.5 to 8.5% with an average of 3.8%. In Anchuthengu $CaCO_3$ ranges from 0.3 to 20.8 % with an average of 4.56% ranges from 0.25 to 6.83 % with an average of 4.6%. In Kappil-Hariharapuram $CaCO_3$ % samples ranges from 1.0 to 11.5 % with an average of 5.8%. $CaCO_3$ % in the Kayamkulam sediments of ranges from 0.5 to 21.5 % with an average of 4.5%. It is due to abundance of silty substrates. Elevated percentages of calcium carboante content reported at the estuary is due to the leaching of shelled organisms. The high values of $CaCO_3$ in sediment sample is mainly due to shell fragments, while lower $CaCO_3$ suggest the active detritus dilution, which has reduced the concentration of $CaCO_3$.

The majority of the organic content in the sediments comes from marine or land plants, or both. The rate of accumulation of organic and inorganic matter, as well as the rate of organic matter decomposition after deposition, determine the rate of sedimentary organic matter. In other words, organic matter plays a major role in concentrating trace metals. In the Kadinamkulam estuary, the organic matter content in the sediments ranges from 0.8 to 8.3 % with an average of 4.7%. It is due to abundance of silt and mangrove remains. In Anchuthengu estuary, it ranges from 0.9 to 6.8 % with an average of 3.0%. The maximum concentration of OM% is seen in the northern part of the estuary, is due to the higher terrigenous materials input and untreated sewage discharge from nearby urbanised regions. The organic matter content in the sediments of Kappil-Hariharapuram estuary ranges from 0.2 to 8.6 % with an average of 3.3%. The low OM% in the estuay is due to the constant influence of freshwater. The organic matter content in the Kayamkulam estuarine sediments of ranges from 0.3 to 13.7 % with an average of 5.9%. Higher percentages of OM is due to abundance of silt and mangrove remains. Slightly higher concentrations observed in the surface samples may be due to the adsorption and incorporation of organic materials from overlying water column. Organic matter in estuarine sediments may be derived from terrestrial, and anthropogenic sources.

## 8.2 ELEMENTAL CONCENTRATION AND POLLUTION INDICES

The results of trace elements of the investigated selected estuarine surface sediments show following decreasing order of its distribution: Kadinamkulam estuary Fe > Cr > Mn > Zn > Ni > Pb > Cu > Co; Anchuthengu estuary Fe > Mn > Cr > Zn > Ni > Pb > Cu > Co; Kappil - Hariharapuram Fe > Mn > Cr > Zn > Cu > Ni > Pb > Co and Kayamkulam estuary Fe > Cr > Mn > Ni > Zn > Pb > Co > Cu. The chief elements occurring in the selected estuarine sediments were Fe and Mn, revealing that they were derived and controlled by the convergence of the terrigenous sources nearer to the estuaries.

The values of EF in the selected estuaries in the following decreasing order Cr > Pb > Mn > Cu > Zn > Ni > Co for Kadinamkulam estuary, Cr >Pb >Mn > Cu > Ni >Zn > Co for Anchuthengu estuary, Cr > Pb > Cu > Mn > Zn > Ni > Co for Kappil - Hariharapuram estuary and Cr > Pb > Mn > Ni > Zn > Co > Cu for Kayamkulam estuary respectively. All of the metal enrichment in this investigation was found to be natural enrichment to severe enrichment. The above-mentioned metal enrichment trend shows natural to extremely severe enrichment in the estuarine sediments derived from the geogenic process to severe anthropogenic influences, whereas Pb and Cr showing moderately severe to severe enrichment. These two metals infer their origin is from anthropogenic sources such as atmospheric deposition, fishing activities and anti-fouling agents used as coatings in boats. Significant enrichment of Pb controls over many trace elements is evident. From the obtained results of Pb, shows severe enrichment which may have partly originated from anthropogenic sources, such as fisheries, extensive use of antifouling and anticorrosive paints by shipping activities, ship wastes, and atmospheric deposits.

The contamination factor of the investigated selected estuarine surface sediments shows following decreasing order of its distribution: Kadinamkulam estuary Cr > Pb > Mn > Zn > Cu > Ni > Fe > Co; Anchuthengu estuary Cr > Pb > Mn > Cu > Zn > Ni > Fe > Co; Kappil – Hariharapuram estuary Cr > Pb > Cu > Mn > Zn > Ni > Fe > Co and Kayamkulam estuary Cr > Pb > Mn > Ni > Zn > Co > Fe > Cu. The most dominant trace elements contaminating sediments in the four estuaries are Cr and Pb. Most probably these elements are derived from several activities of thermal power plant, fisheries and atmospheric deposition along the estuaries and coast. The level of contamination for the selected estuaries was observed by lead and chromium to the very high contamination degree, whereas the other elements show moderate to considerable degree of contamination.

The results of the geo-accumulation index are found to be variating from unpolluted to extremely polluted and that too changing from location to location and also metal to metal, in all four estuaries. The mean of the $I_{geo}$ values of the sediments was moderately to strongly polluted by Cr and Pb in Kadinamkulam estuary and Anchuthengu estuary; by Cr, Pb, Cu and Mn in Kappil-Hariharapuram estuary. and by Cr, Pb and Mn in Kayamkulam estuary. Whereas the sediments were unpolluted to moderately polluted by other metals like Fe, Co, Ni and Zn in all the four estuaries.

The PLI of the studied estuaries ranging from 1.23 to 5.42 in Kadinamkulam estuary indicating sediments were polluted by the metal concentration, PLI ranging from 2.48 to 7.30 in Anchuthengu estuary indicating the sediments were polluted by the metal concentration, PLI

Department of Geology, UNOM

values of all the sediments in Kappil- Hariharapuram estuary and Kayamkulam estuary exceeding 1 indicating pollution by the metal concentration. Anthropogenic influences majorly control the levels of PLI of the sediments. The investigation show pollution in all the samples with that it is concluded the present environment is considered to be polluted based on the PLI study.

The investigation based on the SPI shows that sediments in Kadinamkulam estuary ranges from natural sediments to moderately polluted sediments, in Anchuthengu estuary SPI values ranges from low polluted to moderately polluted sediments, in Kappil- Hariharapuram estuary SPI value ranges from moderately polluted to highly polluted sediments and in Kayamkulam estuary the SPI value ranges from moderately polluted to highly polluted sediments.

The level of potential ecological risk ranges from 44.96 to 126.42 in Kadinamkulam estuary with a mean value of 104.59; 65.53 to 165.78 in Anchuthengu estuary with a mean value of 108.48; 93.1 to 272.71 with an average of 143.43 in Kappil – Hariharapuram estuary and 86.80 to 211.96 with an average of 112.62 in Kayamkulam estuary. The grades of ecological risk of the metals suggest that all the elements fall under the low-risk category in Kadinamkulam estuary, 3 samples falling under moderately risk and all remaining samples under low-risk category in Anchuthengu estuary; 7 samples falling under moderately risk and all other samples under low-risk category in Kappil – Hariharapuram estuary and 2 samples falling under moderately risk and all other samples under low-risk category in Kayamkulam estuary.

## 8.3 MICROPLASTICS (MPs)

The overall microplastics were dominated by coloured plastics (79.01%) followed by white coloured plastics (20.99%). The size and shape classification suggest that they are conquered by < 1000 μm and fibre shape microplastic, respectively. The estuarine sediments were dominated by polyester (49.88), polyethylene (36.36%) followed by polypropylene (13.76%). The mean abundance of the microplastic distribution in the sediments of selected estuaries was 628 particles/kg. The occurrence of the microplastic in sediments was due to the proximity of urban regions, distance of the sampling point from the coast. The FTIR studies revealed that polyethylene, polyester and polypropylene were the dominant polymers among different types of microplastics in estuarine surface sediments. The proper solid waste management, adoption of correct policies and creation of the awareness among the people the negative impact of microplastic to the environment may be the solution for this problem.

The combined use of PHI and PERI in this work offered a preliminary ecological risk assessment induced by MP contamination in selected estuary sediments along Kerala's south coast. The overall risk of MP pollution in present study was categorized as Hazard level IV to V, based on PHI values. Due to the existence of MPs with high hazard scores, which including PA and PS, the PHI values of Kadinamkulam are high (>1000). In Kappil-Hariharapuram (S. no. 56), (S.no. 81) two samples and Kayamkulam estuary two samples (S.no. 99 and 101) have values lesser than 1000 falling under PHI category IV respectively. Apart from these four samples, all the other samples in the analyzed estuarine sediments falling under the PHI category V. The potential ecological risk index (PERI) values of selected estuarine sediments of the present study display extreme ecological risk (PERI: >1200) from collective MP polymers in sediments from Kadinamkulam, Anchuthengu, Kappil- Hariharapuram and Kayamkulam estuaries.

## 8.4 POLYCYCLIC AROMATIC HYDROCARBONS (PAHs)

The analytical results of PAHs concluded that the surface sediments of the selected estuarine system falling under the low contamination and low-risk category. PAH sources can be identified using the ratio of low molecular weight to high molecular weight PAH components. The estimated ratio >1 denotes a petrogenic source of PAH, whereas the ratio <1 denotes a pyrolytic source. The ratio of LMW/HMW PAHs in this study indicates that pyrolytic fractions predominate in these estuaries. Furthermore, the current study region was less polluted by polycyclic aromatic hydrocarbons (PAHs) and posed less of an ecological risk. When compared to other study regions throughout the world, the concentration of PAHs in selected estuaries on the west coast was lower.

## 8.5 OVERALL ECOLOGICAL RISK ASSESSMENT OF THE SELECTED ESTUARY

The investigation concludes that the present study environment is considered to be polluted based on the PLI study. Anthropogenic impacts chiefly control the levels of PLI of the sediments. The study based on the SPI shows that sediments in selected estuaries ranges from natural sediments to highly polluted sediments. With majority of the sediments falling under the category moderately polluted sediments. The grades of ecological risk of the metals suggest that in the

Department of Geology, UNOM

selected estuaries majority of the sediment fall under the low-risk category. Further, the current study location was also less polluted by polycyclic aromatic hydrocarbons (PAHs) and posed a lower risk to the environment.

The potential ecological risk index (PERI) values of selected estuaries show extreme ecological risk from combined MP polymers in sediments from Kadinamkulam, Anchuthengu, Kappil- Hariharapuram and Kayamkulam. Since PERI is evaluated based on the hazard score since toxicity score for PS are high, and as a result, the highest PERI was noted. Although there is no discernible relationship between MP abundance and PHI based on the observations gathered, increasing MP abundance may pose an ecological risk.

Various persistent pollutants such as trace elements, microplastics and PAHs were subjected to determine the ecological risk status from the sediments in the selected estuaries of the south west coast of Kerala, India. Based on the results from these proxies, the overall risk status for the ecology of the selected estuaries is falling in low-risk status. However, risk status based on microplastics show extreme risk since the toxicity scores and the calculations involving are not yet formulated and well standardised since the toxicity calculations of microplastics is an emerging study.

## 8.6 RECOMMENDATIONS

This research aids future evaluations of the interaction between anthropogenic effect and organisms. This finding could be crucial for future efforts to conserve and manage the estuary environment. Since these contaminants are falling under the emerging contaminants category and persistent pollutants category, there is an utmost necessity to focus and monitor these pollutants very carefully. Even nano level of its presence will be harmful and have adverse effect on the environment compartments. For several of these pollutants do not have any standard limit or threshold limit by various organizations, so these pollutants should be monitored very carefully in upcoming years.

CPSIA information can be obtained
at www.ICGtesting.com
Printed in the USA
BVHW051421110423
662129BV00011B/960

9 781805 253105